SpringerBriefs in Genetics

C000048799

For further volumes:
http://www.springer.com/series/8923

C. Alexander Valencia • M. Ali Pervaiz
Ammar Husami • Yaping Qian • Kejian Zhang

Next Generation Sequencing Technologies in Medical Genetics

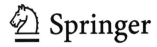 Springer

C. Alexander Valencia
Division of Human Genetics
Cincinnati Children's Hospital
    Medical Center
Cincinnati, OH, USA

Ammar Husami
Division of Human Genetics
Cincinnati Children's Hospital
    Medical Center
Cincinnati, OH, USA

Kejian Zhang
Division of Human Genetics
Cincinnati Children's Hospital
    Medical Center
Cincinnati, OH, USA

M. Ali Pervaiz
WellStar Douglas Hospital
WellStar Health System
Douglasville, GA, USA

Yaping Qian
Division of Human Genetics
Cincinnati Children's Hospital
    Medical Center
Cincinnati, OH, USA

ISSN 2191-5563   ISSN 2191-5571 (electronic)
ISBN 978-1-4614-9031-9   ISBN 978-1-4614-9032-6 (eBook)
DOI 10.1007/978-1-4614-9032-6
Springer New York Heidelberg Dordrecht London

Library of Congress Control Number: 2013949287

Springer is part of Springer Science+Business Media (www.springer.com)

Preface

The purpose of this book is to serve as an introduction to those that want to learn about next-generation–sequencing (NGS) and its applications. However, from the middle to end of each chapter a more in-depth approach will be taken to satisfy the curious minds of professionals in the fields of medical genetics and other related disciplines. Most chapters will contain one figure or table illustrating principles or summarizing key findings in the field.

A book search on Amazon and Google on "next-generation–sequencing" leads to book hits covering a wide range of topics including (1) NGS methods, (2) NGS informatics, (3) application to microRNA expression profiling, (4) application to personalize medicine, (5) application to plant sciences, and (6) challenges and opportunities of NGS for biomedical research. However, none of these books describes the direct application of NGS to medicine, specifically, laboratory medicine or molecular diagnostics. This book will bridge the gap between research and direct application to patient care. I foresee this book as the first, of many to come, translation medicine books in this field. Moreover, being a part of the Briefs in Genetic series will allow the reader to quickly become familiar with the technologies and most importantly their clinical applications. Furthermore, throughout the book the recent developments are briefly summarized.

In this book (Part I), we introduce the reader to the wealth of next-generation technologies followed by their direct applications (Part II) in the diagnosis of genetic disorders in the field broadly known as medical genetics. We will separate Parts I and II equally because this will allow a more in-depth description of the technologies for those that require a more profound understanding of the technologies. The equal space split, Part II, will provide the opportunity to describe the applications of NGS to molecular diagnostics by starting with a comprehensive view of the genetic disorders that have been analyzed by these technologies and then we focus on several of these genetic disorder examples including muscular dystrophy and hearing loss. Within these disorder-based chapters, we will describe the disorder and how NGS has been an excellent tool for reaching a diagnosis of previously undiagnosed patients. Furthermore, we will discuss the additional NGS benefits, namely, increased sequencing throughput and decreased cost that patients can obtain from these tests. It can be speculated that NGS will become an even more popular platform in laboratory medicine and it can be argued that the technology is here to stay to provide better patient care by reaching a diagnosis sooner. Finally, we will end the book by briefly acknowledging the breakthroughs, in light of eight other chapters that describe the triumphs of the technologies, and focus on the challenges that lie ahead and suggest possible solutions to such challenges.

Cincinnati, OH   C. Alexander Valencia
                                                                                          Ammar Husami
                                                                                             Yaping Qian
                                                                                            Kejian Zhang
Douglasville, GA   M. Ali Pervaiz

Acknowledgements

I would like to take this opportunity to thank all contributors of this book. It was a great pleasure and an enjoyable experience working with you on this project.

I would like to express my gratitude to the many people who provided support, talked things over, read, offered comments, and assisted in the proofreading.

This book is dedicated to our families, who supported and encouraged us in spite of all the time it took me away from them.

C. Alexander Valencia, Ph.D.

Contents

Part I
Advances in Next-Generation–Sequencing Technology

Chapter 1
Sanger Sequencing Principles, History, and Landmarks

1.1 Historical Overview

The first DNA sequencing (1968) was performed 15 years after the discovery of the double helix (1953) (Hutchison 2007). However, the chemical method of Maxam and Gilbert and the dideoxy method of Sanger began in the mid-1970s (Fig. 1.1). The profound insights into genetic organization were shown by Nicklen and Coulson with the first complete DNA sequence of phage ϕX174. As sequencing output improved, larger molecules greater than 200 kb (human cytomegalovirus) were sequenced and computational analysis and bioinformatics was born. Sequencing efforts reached new heights with the initiation of the US Human Genome Project culminating in the first "sequencing factory" by 1992 (Hutchison 2007). With this effort came the sequencing of the first bacterial genome, by 1995, and other small eubacterial, archaebacterial, and eukaryotic genomes soon thereafter. Published in 2001, the working draft of the human genome sequence was the result of the competition between the public Human Genome Project and Celera Genomics (Fig. 1.1). The new "massively parallel" sequencing methods (Chap. 2) are greatly increasing sequencing capacity, but further innovations are needed to achieve the "thousand dollar genome" that many feel is the prerequisite to personalized genomic medicine (Fig. 1.1). These advances will also allow new approaches to a variety of problems in biology, evolution, and the environment.

In this chapter we describe the principles and history of Sanger sequencing that led to the creation of sequencing centers that were eventually responsible for sequencing the human genome, the dawn of genomic medicine. In addition, we briefly introduce the principle and platforms available for NGS and conclude by reflecting on the dream of achieving the $1,000 genome through computational support. Moreover, in Part I of this book (Chaps. 1, 2, and 3), we will discuss in detail the principles of next-generation–sequencing (NGS; Chap. 2) and enrichment technologies (Chap. 3). In Part II, we will include the clinical applications of NGS in medical genetics. Specifically, a cursory view of the field will be covered (Chap. 4),

C.A. Valencia et al., *Next Generation Sequencing Technologies in Medical Genetics*,
SpringerBriefs in Genetics, DOI 10.1007/978-1-4614-9032-6_1,
© C. Alexander Valencia 2013

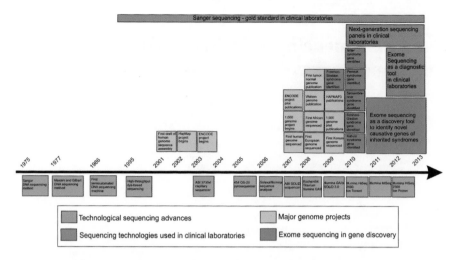

Fig. 1.1 Timeline of the major advances in sequencing technologies starting with Sanger sequencing and ending with the next-generation–sequencing (*blue*). The major genome projects that were made possible by these methods are shown (*yellow*). In addition to clinical exome sequencing, the timeline of Sanger sequencing as a gold standard in clinical laboratories is depicted (*purple*). The uses of NGS in exome sequencing project with gene discovery objectives have also been noted (*green*)

followed by specific genetic disorder examples where NGS technologies have made great advancement in the diagnosis of patients including prenatal diagnosis (Chap. 5), muscular dystrophies (Chap. 6), hearing loss (Chap. 7), and exome analysis as applied to gene discovery and molecular diagnostics (Chap. 8). There are advantages and disadvantages to all technologies. In Chap. 9, we will address the challenges of NGS in molecular diagnostics.

1.2   Principle of Sanger Sequencing

In 1975, Sanger introduced his "plus and minus" method for DNA sequencing (Fig. 1.1; Sanger and Coulson 1975). This was a critical transition technique leading to the modern generation of methods that have completely dominated sequencing over the past 30 years. The key to this advance was the use of polyacrylamide gels to separate the products of primed synthesis by DNA polymerase in order of increasing chain length (Hutchison 2007). In Sanger dideoxy DNA sequencing, a DNA-dependent polymerase is used to generate a complimentary copy of a single-stranded DNA template, also known as sequencing by synthesis (SBS) (Sanger 1988; Sanger et al. 1977a, b). By beginning at the 3′ end, a new chain of a primer DNA complementary to a single-stranded "template" DNA strand is synthesized.

At this time, the deoxynucleotides are added to the growing chain and are complementary to the nucleotides in the template DNA. The creation of a phosphodiester bridge between the 3′ hydroxyl group at the growing end of the primer and the 5′ phosphate group of the incoming deoxynucleotide elongates the DNA chain, with the corresponding dNTP releasing pyrophosphate (PPi) when a dNMP is incorporated (Shendure et al. 2011).

The original dideoxy chain termination DNA sequencing technology utilizes the fact that DNA polymerases will incorporate a chain-terminating 2′,3′-dideoxynucleotide monophosphate (ddNMP) at the appropriate complementary position but synthesis will be stopped by the incorporation of the ddNMPs at the 3′ end because the next nucleotide to be added lacks the required 3′ hydroxyl group for dNMP phosphodiester bond formation (Sanger et al. 1977b; Shendure et al. 2011). Four reactions, containing template, polymerase, all four dNTPs (one radioactively labeled), and primer, are set up to generate a continuing series of synthesis products that reflects each potential chain termination position. In addition, each reaction also contains one of the four ddNTPs at a specific ratio reflecting the relative probability of incorporation. Many terminated strands of different lengths exist within each of the four reactions. As each reaction contains only one ddNTP species, a set of different-length fragments is generated in each reaction, terminated at all of the positions corresponding to one of the four nucleotides in the template sequence. The four reactions are then individually separated on a large denaturing polyacrylamide gel to yield single-nucleotide resolution. The pattern of bands across the four lanes allows direct readout of the primary sequence of the template under analysis.

The original radioactive Sanger dideoxy sequencing protocols, which used [α-^{32}P]dATP to label the growing DNA chains, were modified to use [α-^{35}S]dATP or [α-^{33}P]dATP because the lower-energy β emissions of ^{35}S and ^{33}P result in sharper autoradiographic bands, allowing more (longer) sequence to be read (Shendure et al. 2011). Sequences generated using [α-^{33}P]dATP have short exposure times similar to ^{32}P, but band resolution comparable to that of ^{35}S (Zagursky et al. 1991). Another advantage of using ^{33}P and ^{35}S is that users are exposed to lower radiation doses than with ^{32}P. In lieu of using radioactivity, a chemiluminescent detection method was developed that is comparable in sensitivity to traditional radiolabeling. A biotinylated primer is used in the dideoxy sequencing reactions and, after electrophoresis of the biotinylated sequencing products on a sequencing gel, the products are transferred from the gel to a nylon membrane. After UV cross-linking the DNA to the membrane, the membrane is treated with streptavidin, biotinylated alkaline phosphatase, and a detection reagent, such as CDP* (Tropix/Applied Biosystems), which emits light upon dephosphorylation. After exposure to X-ray film, the resultant lumigram can be read in a manner similar to an autoradiogram when using radioactivity (Beck et al. 1989; Creasey et al. 1991; Tizard et al. 1990). Technology for end labeling of DNA fragments with biotin allowed this detection method to also be used in chemical sequencing reactions (Tizard et al. 1990).

1.3   First-Generation Automated Sanger DNA Sequencing

Toward the end of the manual-sequencing era, in 1986 the first generation of "automated sequencers," pioneered by Applied BioSystems (now part of Life Technologies), appeared and included automation of the gel electrophoresis steps, detection of the fluorescent DNA band patterns, and analysis of bands (Fig. 1.1; Smith et al. 1986). The four sets of sequencing reactions were loaded onto slab gels manually and electrophoresis automated. The sequence was obtained by recording the moving bands sequentially past a detector at the bottom of the gel. The replacement of radioactivity with fluorescently labeled primers or ddNTPs and development of polymerases that could effectively incorporate these dyes were essential to the automation process and this remains the general method of choice for these first-generation automated DNA sequencers. Today, automated DNA sequencing performed today makes use of automated capillary electrophoresis, which typically analyzes 8–96 sequencing reactions simultaneously, in combination with the use of the latest generation of fluorescent dyes that exhibit strong and distinct fluorescent emissions (Fig. 1.1; Ju et al. 1996). Thus, implementations of "first-generation automated DNA sequencing" had key advantages over methods described for the original Sanger sequencing, namely, the elimination of radioactivity use, "one-lane" sequencing, "one-tube" reactions, automated base calling, and elimination of slab-gel technology in favor of multi-capillary electrophoresis with automatic, electrokinetic-injection lane loading.

1.4   Automated Sequencing Factories

Craig Venter and colleagues at NIH used the ABI 370A DNA sequencer to determine the sequence of a gene (Gocayne et al. 1987). At NIH, Venter set up a sequencing facility containing six automated sequencers and two ABI Catalyst robots. In 1992, Venter established The Institute for Genomic Research (TIGR) to expand his sequencing operation with 30 ABI 373A automated sequencers and 17 ABI Catalyst 800 robots (Adams et al. 1994). This was a real factory with teams dedicated to different steps in the sequencing process such as template preparation, gel pouring, and sequencer operation. Data analysis was integrated into the process so that problems in earlier steps could be detected and corrected as soon as possible.

An early demonstration of the power of automated sequencing was the development of the expressed sequence tag (EST) approach to gene discovery. In this approach, cDNA copies of messenger RNA were cloned at random and subjected to automated sequencing. In the first report from Venter and colleagues in 1991, 337 new human genes were reported, 48 homologous to genes from other organisms (Adams et al. 1991). This approach was adopted by many genome projects. Today, the EST database contains over 43 million ESTs from over 1,300 different organisms. Another early application of the automated sequencer was the worm genome sequencing project which was underway by 1992 with the beginning elements of a factory atmosphere as well (Sulston et al. 1992). In 1993 the Sanger Centre, later renamed the Wellcome Trust Sanger Institute, was established by the Wellcome Trust and the Medical Research Council. The facility has produced ~3.4×10^9 bases of finished sequence by the 30th anniversary of the dideoxy sequencing method.

1.5 Sequencing the Human Genome

Eventually, sequencing of the human genome became an imaginable goal at the outset of the sequencing era 30 years ago. Formal discussions of the idea began in 1985 when Robert Sinsheimer organized a meeting on human genome sequencing at the University of California, Santa Cruz (Sinsheimer 2006). That same year Charles DeLisi and David A. Smith commissioned the first Santa Fe conference, funded by the DOE, to study the feasibility of a Human Genome Initiative. In 1990 the DOE and NIH presented a joint 5-year US Human Genome Project plan to Congress. It was estimated that the project would take 15 years and cost ~3 billion US$ (Fig. 1.1).

The US Human Genome Project established goals of mapping, and in some cases sequencing, several model organisms as well as humans. These included *E. coli*, yeast (*S. cerevisiae*), the worm (*C. elegans*), drosophila (*D. melanogaster*), and mouse (laboratory strains of *Mus domesticus*). The publicly funded effort became an international collaboration between a number of sequencing centers in the United States, Europe, and Japan. Each center focused sequencing efforts on particular regions of the genome, necessitating detailed mapping as a first step. In 1994, a detailed genetic map of the human genome was published including 5,840 mapped loci (Murray et al. 1994). In 1998 the public project, now in a race with Celera, also adopted the new ABI Prism 3700 capillary sequencers. In 1999 the Human Genome Project celebrated passing the billion base-pair mark, and the first complete sequence of a human chromosome was reported [chromosome 22] (Dunham et al. 1999). On 25 June 2000 at the White House, President Clinton with Prime Minister Tony Blair publicly announced draft versions of the human genome sequence from both the publicly funded project and from Celera (Fig. 1.1). In February 2001, the Celera and the public draft human genome sequences were published the same week in Science and Nature (Lander et al. 2001; Venter et al. 2001).

1.6 Overview of Next-Generation–Sequencing and Clinical Applications

In the last few years, methods have emerged that challenge the gold standard of dideoxy Sanger sequencing. All of these recently developed non-Sanger commercial sequencing platforms, including systems from 454/Roche, Illumina, Applied Biosystems/Life Technologies, Dover, Helicos Biosciences, Ion Torrent, and Ion

Proton (now part of Life Technologies), fall under the rubric of a single paradigm termed cyclic array sequencing (Chap. 2; Fig. 1.1; Metzker 2010). Cyclic array platforms achieve low costs by "massively parallel" sequencing, meaning that the number of sequence reads from a single experiment is vastly greater than the 96 obtained with modern capillary electrophoresis-based Sanger sequencers. At present this very high throughput is achieved with substantial sacrifices in length and accuracy of the individual reads when compared to Sanger sequencing. Nonetheless, assemblies of such data can be highly accurate because of the high degree of sequence coverage obtainable. They are most readily applied to sequencing, in which sequence data is aligned with a reference genome sequence in order to look for differences from that reference. A few examples of enrichment and NGS sequencing technologies are discussed in Chaps. 2 and 3, respectively. Other technologies are under development and all of these methods will undoubtedly continue to improve.

Within the last 5 years, high-throughput sequencing technologies have successfully identified mutations in novel genes for a number of genetic conditions, including Sensenbrenner syndrome, Kabuki syndrome, and Miller syndrome (Fig. 1.1; Gilissen et al. 2010; Ng et al. 2010). NGS facilitates target sequencing for rapid, accurate, and lower cost diagnostic applications. However, with several target enrichment strategies, including microarray-based capture, in-solution capture, and polymerase chain reaction (PCR)-based amplification (Albert et al. 2007; Gnirke et al. 2009; Hodges et al. 2007, 2009; Kirkness 2009; Nikolaev et al. 2009; Okou et al. 2007; Tewhey et al. 2009), and NGS sequencing platforms, selection and validation of the technologies becomes crucial for clinical applications (Metzker 2010; Voelkerding et al. 2009). In the last 2 years, a number of clinical NGS panels have been developed for mutation detection of genes in a number of phenotypic and/or genetically heterogeneous disorders including muscular dystrophies and hearing loss (Schrauwen et al. 2013; Sivakumaran et al. 2013; Valencia et al. 2012, 2013). Moreover, three large-scale clinical studies were published showing results that NGS of maternal DNA of pregnant women is a powerful molecular diagnostic tool for diagnosis of fetal aneuploidies (Chiu et al. 2011; Ehrich et al. 2011; Palomaki et al. 2011). The clinical applications are discussed in more detail in Part II, Chaps. 4, 5, 6, 7, 8, and 9, of this book.

1.7   Future Trends

In the coming years, molecular diagnostics will continue to be of critical importance to public health worldwide. Molecular genetic testing will facilitate the detection and characterization of disease, as well as monitoring of drug response, and will assist in the identification of genetic modifiers and disease susceptibility. Massively parallel methods are likely to dominate clinical high-throughput sequencing applications for the next few years. However, a variety of other approaches are being investigated that may eventually be developed into practical methods (Chan 2005).

Regardless of the method, exons with highly repetitive and high GC regions are not well enriched and will require Sanger sequencing for completeness and confirmatory testing (Valencia et al. 2012).

The currently popular vision that a clinical laboratory with a single benchtop machine could replace a large sequencing center can only be realized with increases in the productivity of computers and bioinformaticians even more dramatic than that expected for sequencers. It appears that for an individual $1,000 genome sequences to be truly useful, fundamental advances in computation and bioinformatics will be essential for data handling, storage, and interpretation. The obvious importance of computational analysis of sequence data has led to a greater overall appreciation of the role of theory in biology. A relationship between theory and experiment, not unlike that found in the twentieth century physics, seems to be taking shape.

References

Adams MD, Kelley JM, Gocayne JD et al (1991) Complementary DNA sequencing: expressed sequence tags and human genome project. Science 252:1651–1656

Adams MD, Kerlavage AR, Kelley JM et al (1994) A model for high-throughput automated DNA sequencing and analysis core facilities. Nature 368:474–475. doi:10.1038/368474a0

Albert TJ, Molla MN, Muzny DM et al (2007) Direct selection of human genomic loci by microarray hybridization. Nat Methods 4:903–905. doi:10.1038/nmeth1111

Beck S, O'Keeffe T, Coull JM, Köster H (1989) Chemiluminescent detection of DNA: application for DNA sequencing and hybridization. Nucleic Acids Res 17:5115–5123

Chan EY (2005) Advances in sequencing technology. Mutat Res 573:13–40. doi:10.1016/j.mrfmmm.2005.01.004

Chiu RWK, Akolekar R, Zheng YWL et al (2011) Non-invasive prenatal assessment of trisomy 21 by multiplexed maternal plasma DNA sequencing: large scale validity study. BMJ 342:c7401

Creasey A, D'Angio L Jr, Dunne TS et al (1991) Application of a novel chemiluminescence-based DNA detection method to single-vector and multiplex DNA sequencing. BioTechniques 11:102–104, 106, 108–109

Dunham I, Shimizu N, Roe BA et al (1999) The DNA sequence of human chromosome 22. Nature 402:489–495. doi:10.1038/990031

Ehrich M, Deciu C, Zwiefelhofer T et al (2011) Noninvasive detection of fetal trisomy 21 by sequencing of DNA in maternal blood: a study in a clinical setting. Am J Obstet Gynecol 204:205.e1–205.e11. doi:10.1016/j.ajog.2010.12.060

Gilissen C, Arts HH, Hoischen A et al (2010) Exome sequencing identifies WDR35 variants involved in Sensenbrenner syndrome. Am J Hum Genet 87:418–423. doi:10.1016/j.ajhg.2010.08.004

Gnirke A, Melnikov A, Maguire J et al (2009) Solution hybrid selection with ultra-long oligonucleotides for massively parallel targeted sequencing. Nat Biotechnol 27:182–189. doi:10.1038/nbt.1523

Gocayne J, Robinson DA, FitzGerald MG et al (1987) Primary structure of rat cardiac beta-adrenergic and muscarinic cholinergic receptors obtained by automated DNA sequence analysis: further evidence for a multigene family. Proc Natl Acad Sci U S A 84:8296–8300

Hodges E, Xuan Z, Balija V et al (2007) Genome-wide in situ exon capture for selective resequencing. Nat Genet 39:1522–1527. doi:10.1038/ng.2007.42

Hodges E, Rooks M, Xuan Z et al (2009) Hybrid selection of discrete genomic intervals on custom-designed microarrays for massively parallel sequencing. Nat Protoc 4:960–974. doi:10.1038/nprot.2009.68

Hutchison CA 3rd (2007) DNA sequencing: bench to bedside and beyond. Nucleic Acids Res 35:6227–6237. doi:10.1093/nar/gkm688

Ju J, Glazer AN, Mathies RA (1996) Energy transfer primers: a new fluorescence labeling paradigm for DNA sequencing and analysis. Nat Med 2:246–249

Kirkness EF (2009) Targeted sequencing with microfluidics. Nat Biotechnol 27:998–999. doi:10.1038/nbt1109-998

Lander ES, Linton LM, Birren B et al (2001) Initial sequencing and analysis of the human genome. Nature 409:860–921. doi:10.1038/35057062

Metzker ML (2010) Sequencing technologies—the next-generation generation. Nat Rev Genet 11:31–46. doi:10.1038/nrg2626

Murray JC, Buetow KH, Weber JL et al (1994) A comprehensive human linkage map with centimorgan density. Cooperative Human Linkage Center (CHLC). Science 265:2049–2054

Ng SB, Bigham AW, Buckingham KJ et al (2010) Exome sequencing identifies MLL2 mutations as a cause of Kabuki syndrome. Nat Genet 42:790–793. doi:10.1038/ng.646

Nikolaev SI, Iseli C, Sharp AJ et al (2009) Detection of genomic variation by selection of a 9 mb DNA region and high throughput sequencing. PLoS One 4:e6659. doi:10.1371/journal.pone.0006659

Okou DT, Steinberg KM, Middle C et al (2007) Microarray-based genomic selection for high-throughput resequencing. Nat Methods 4:907–909. doi:10.1038/nmeth1109

Palomaki GE, Kloza EM, Lambert-Messerlian GM et al (2011) DNA sequencing of maternal plasma to detect Down syndrome: an international clinical validation study. Genet Med 13:913–920. doi:10.1097/GIM.0b013e3182368a0e

Sanger F (1988) Sequences, sequences, and sequences. Annu Rev Biochem 57:1–28. doi:10.1146/annurev.bi.57.070188.000245

Sanger F, Coulson AR (1975) A rapid method for determining sequences in DNA by primed synthesis with DNA polymerase. J Mol Biol 94:441–448

Sanger F, Air GM, Barrell BG et al (1977a) Nucleotide sequence of bacteriophage phi X174 DNA. Nature 265:687–695

Sanger F, Nicklen S, Coulson AR (1977b) DNA sequencing with chain-terminating inhibitors. Proc Natl Acad Sci U S A 74:5463–5467

Schrauwen I, Sommen M, Corneveaux JJ et al (2013) A sensitive and specific diagnostic test for hearing loss using a microdroplet PCR-based approach and next-generation sequencing. Am J Med Genet A 161A:145–152. doi:10.1002/ajmg.a.35737

Shendure JA, Porreca GJ, Church GM et al (2011) Overview of DNA sequencing strategies. In: FM Ausubel et al (ed) Curr Protoc Mol Biol, Chapter 7, Unit 7.1. John Wiley & Sons, Inc. doi:10.1002/0471142727.mb0701s96

Sinsheimer RL (2006) To reveal the genomes. Am J Hum Genet 79:194–196. doi:10.1086/505887

Sivakumaran TA, Husami A, Kissell D et al (2013) Performance evaluation of the next-generation sequencing approach for molecular diagnosis of hereditary hearing loss. Otolaryngol Head Neck Surg. doi:10.1177/0194599813482294

Smith LM, Sanders JZ, Kaiser RJ et al (1986) Fluorescence detection in automated DNA sequence analysis. Nature 321:674–679. doi:10.1038/321674a0

Sulston J, Du Z, Thomas K et al (1992) The C. elegans genome sequencing project: a beginning. Nature 356:37–41. doi:10.1038/356037a0

Tewhey R, Warner JB, Nakano M et al (2009) Microdroplet-based PCR enrichment for large-scale targeted sequencing. Nat Biotechnol 27:1025–1031. doi:10.1038/nbt.1583

Tizard R, Cate RL, Ramachandran KL et al (1990) Imaging of DNA sequences with chemiluminescence. Proc Natl Acad Sci U S A 87:4514–4518

Valencia CA, Rhodenizer D, Bhide S et al (2012) Assessment of target enrichment platforms using massively parallel sequencing for the mutation detection for congenital muscular dystrophy. J Mol Diagn 14:233–246. doi:10.1016/j.jmoldx.2012.01.009

Valencia CA, Ankala A, Rhodenizer D et al (2013) Comprehensive mutation analysis for congenital muscular dystrophy: a clinical PCR-based enrichment and next-generation sequencing panel. PLoS One 8:e53083. doi:10.1371/journal.pone.0053083

Venter JC, Adams MD, Myers EW et al (2001) The sequence of the human genome. Science 291:1304–1351. doi:10.1126/science.1058040

Voelkerding KV, Dames SA, Durtschi JD (2009) Next-generation sequencing: from basic research to diagnostics. Clin Chem 55:641–658. doi:10.1373/clinchem.2008.112789

Zagursky RJ, Conway PS, Kashdan MA (1991) Use of 33P for Sanger DNA sequencing. Biotechniques 11(36):38

Chapter 2
A Survey of Next-Generation–Sequencing Technologies

2.1 Introduction

Innovative application of new technologies in research is one of the major factors driving advances in knowledge acquisition. In 1977, Maxam and Gilbert reported an approach in which terminally labeled DNA fragments were subjected to base-specific chemical cleavage and the reaction products were separated by gel electrophoresis (Maxam and Gilbert 1977). In an alternative approach, Sanger described the use of chain-terminating dideoxynucleotide analogs that caused base-specific termination of primed DNA synthesis (Sanger et al. 1977; Chap. 1). Improvements of the Sanger method led to utilization in the research community and eventually in the clinical diagnosis of many genetic disorders (http://www.ncbi.nlm.nih.gov/sites/GeneTests/). In a factory-based format, Sanger sequencing was the method of choice for the first human genome at an estimated cost of $2.7 billion (Fig. 1.1; Chap. 1). In 2008, by comparison, the genome of Dr. James Watson was sequenced over a 2-month period for less than $1 million (Wheeler et al. 2008). With the commercial availability of high-throughput massively parallel DNA sequencing platforms in the past few years, complete sequencing of the whole human genome can be done commercially today in 2–3 months at a cost below $10,000 (Bick and Dimmock 2011; Fig. 1.1). Since their introduction, next-generation–sequencing (NGS) technologies have constantly improved and the costs have steadily decreased. A legitimate question therefore is what role targeted gene capture will play if whole-genome sequencing (WGS) can be done for about $1,000 in the future, with the ability to survey the human genome in an unbiased manner. This chapter describes NGS technologies and briefly explores how they have been translated into molecular diagnostics. The clinical applications of NGS will be covered in detail in Chaps. 4–8.

C.A. Valencia et al., *Next Generation Sequencing Technologies in Medical Genetics*, SpringerBriefs in Genetics, DOI 10.1007/978-1-4614-9032-6_2, © C. Alexander Valencia 2013

Next-generation sequencing workflow

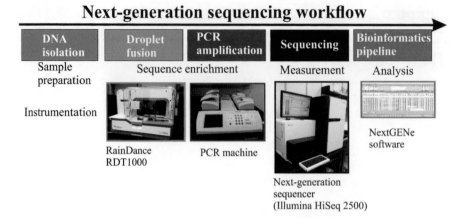

Fig. 2.1 Schematic of the next-generation–sequencing workflow. Following DNA isolation, target sequences are enriched by amplification (RainDance) or capture-based methods, sequenced by a next-generation platform (HiSeq 2500), and analyzed by open source or commercial software package, such as NextGENe from Softgenetics, to obtain the variants that will then be filter prioritized to identify the potentially causative gene(s)

2.2   Fundamentals of NGS Platforms

Generally, NGS is composed of four steps; DNA isolation, target sequences enrichment, sequencing by an NGS platform, and bioinformatic analysis (Fig. 2.1). During the analysis, fragment sequences are aligned and variant calls are obtained and prioritized by applying various filters to identify the potentially causative gene(s). An optional report generation step exists in clinical laboratories after potential causative variants are Sanger-confirmed. A detailed description of the principles and platforms of NGS is mentioned in the next sections.

Massively parallel sequencing is one common feature shared by almost all current NGS platforms, following clonally amplified single DNA molecules, separated in a defined microchamber (called flow cells, flowchips, or picotiter plate; Voelkerding et al. 2009). One exception to this is Pacific Biosciences which uses single-molecule sequencing technology without clonal amplification (Eid et al. 2009). In contrast, Sanger sequencing has orders of magnitude lower throughput by sequencing products produced in individual sequencing reactions. NGS is first carried out by fragmenting the genomic DNA into small pieces, usually in the range of 300–500 bps (Borgström et al. 2011). Then, platform-specific adapters are ligated to the ends of the DNA segments, permitting their attachment and sequencing. In the NGS execution, sequencing results are obtained by reading optical signals during repeated cycles from either polymerase-mediated fluorescent nucleotide extensions of four different colors (e.g., Illumina's HiSeq system), or from iterative cycles of fluorescently labeled oligonucleotide ligation (e.g., ABI

SOLiD system), or by the principle of pyrosequencing (e.g., Roche 454 system; Fig. 1.1; Margulies et al. 2005; Ruparel et al. 2005). Nonoptical DNA sequencing by detecting the hydrogen protons generated by template-directed DNA polymerase synthesis on semiconductor-sensing ion chips has recently been developed as well (Fig. 1.1; Rothberg et al. 2011). In such a massively parallel sequencing process, NGS platforms produce up to 600 Gb of nucleotide sequence from a single instrument run (e.g., Illumina's HiSeq 2000; Clark et al. 2011). The sequenced fragments are called "reads," which could be 25–100 bps from one or both ends. The massive capacity of NGS allows the sequencing of many randomly overlapping DNA fragments; therefore, each nucleotide in targeted regions may be included in many reads, allowing repeated analysis which provides depth of coverage. Increased depth of coverage usually improves sequencing accuracy, because a consensus voting algorithm is used in determining the final nucleotide calls (Lin et al. 2012).

2.3   Roche/454 Life Sciences

Roche 454 utilizes pyrosequencing technology and was the first commercial NGS platform (Fig. 1.1). In contrast to Sanger that uses dideoxynucleotides to terminate the chain amplification, pyrosequencing technology detects the pyrophosphate released during nucleotide incorporation. The library DNAs with 454-specific adapters are denatured into single strands and captured by amplification beads followed by emulsion PCR (Liu et al. 2012). Then on a picotiter plate, one of dNTPs (dATP, dGTP, dCTP, dTTP) will complement the bases of the template strand with the help of ATP sulfurylase, luciferase, luciferin, DNA polymerase, and adenosine 5 phosphosulfate (APS) and release pyrophosphate (PPi) which equals the amount of incorporated nucleotide. The ATP transformed from PPi drives the luciferin into oxyluciferin and generates visible light (Liu et al. 2012). At the same time, the unmatched bases are degraded by apyrase. Then another dNTP is added into the reaction system and the pyrosequencing reaction is repeated.

The read length of Roche 454 was initially 100–150 bp in 2005, 200 K+ reads, and could output 20 Mb per run (Mardis 2008). In 2008, after the launching of the new 454 GS FLX Titanium system, its read length could reach 700 bp with accuracy of 99.9 % and output of 0.7 Gb data per run within 24 h. In 2009, Roche combined the GS Junior a benchtop system into the 454 sequencing system which simplified the library preparation and data processing, and output was also upgraded to 14 Gb per run (Huse et al. 2007). The most notable feature of this system is its run time of approximately 10 h from sequencing to completion. The longer read length is also a distinguishing advantage compared with other NGS systems. In addition, the manpower is reduced by the automation of the library construction and semiautomation of the emulsion PCR. However, the high cost of reagents and the relatively high error rate in terms of polybases longer than 6 bp remain a challenge.

2.4 Illumina/Solexa

In 2006, the Genome Analyzer (GA) became commercially available and was initially released by Solexa and acquired by Illumina in 2007 (Fig. 1.1). In principle, this system obtains sequences by sequencing by synthesis (SBS). The GA uses a flow cell that has an optically transparent slide with eight lanes with surfaces that bind oligonucleotide anchors (Voelkerding et al. 2009). Fragmented template DNA is end-repaired to generate 5′-phosphorylated blunt ends. The adapter oligonucleotides are complementary to the flow-cell anchors. The adapter-modified, single-stranded template DNA is added to the flow cell and immobilized by hybridization to the anchors. DNA templates are amplified in the flow cell by "bridge" amplification resulting in clusters each containing approximately 1,000 clonal molecules. For sequencing, clusters are denatured, chemically cleaved, and washed to leave only forward strands for single-end sequencing. Sequencing of the forward strands is accomplished by primer hybridization complementary to the adapter sequences, addition of polymerase, and by mixing four terminator nucleotides (ddATP, ddGTP, ddCTP, ddTTP) containing a different cleavable fluorescent dye. The terminators are incorporated according to sequence complementarity. After incorporation, excess reagents are washed away, the clusters are optically interrogated, and the fluorescence signal is captured by a charge-coupled device (CCD) (Mardis 2008). With successive chemical steps, the reversible dye terminators are unblocked, the fluorescent labels are cleaved and washed away, and the next sequencing cycle is performed.

Initially, the Solexa GA's output was 1 Gb per run. In 2009, the output of GA increased in three upgrades to 20 Gb per run (75PE), 30 Gb per run (100PE), and 50 Gb per run (150PE), respectively, by improvements in polymerase, buffer, flow cell, and software. The latest GAIIx can reach 85 Gb of sequence per run (Liu et al. 2012). In early 2010, using the same sequencing strategy with GA, Illumina launched the HiSeq 2000 system. The original output of this system was 200 Gb per run and improved to 600 Gb per run which may be completed in 8 days. The error rate of 100PE could be below 2 % on average after filtering. Compared with 454 and Sequencing by Oligo Ligation Detection (SOLiD), HiSeq 2000 provides the lowest cost per million bases ($0.02/Mb). With multiplexing incorporated in P5/P7 primers and adapters, it could handle thousands of samples simultaneously. HiSeq 2000 needs (HiSeq control software) HCS for program control, (real-time analyzer software) RTA to do on-instrument base-calling, and CASAVA for secondary analysis. With the introduction of Truseq v3 reagents and associated software, the HiSeq 2000 instrument can better sequence high GC regions. In 2012, an upgrade to HiSeq 2000 instrument to generate the HiSeq 2500 system was introduced. The HiSeq 2500 system features two run modes, rapid run and high output run, and the ability to process one or two flow cells simultaneously. As with the HiSeq 2000, the HiSeq 2500 in the high output mode can generate 600 Gb per run. However, the HiSeq 2500 has a rapid mode that can generate up to 180 Gb per run in about 40 h. This provides a flexible and scalable platform that supports the broadest range of applications and study sizes.

2.5 Applied Biosystems/SOLiD

The SOLiD system, developed in the laboratory of George Church, was acquired by Applied Biosystems in 2006 (Fig. 1.1). In essence, the sequencer uses short-read sequencing technology by ligation (http://www.solid.appliedbiosystems. com). The resequencing of the *Escherichia coli* genome by SOLiD sequence was reported in 2005 (Shendure et al. 2005). In 2007, Applied Biosystems made improvements to the technology and commercially released the SOLiD instrumentation. Similar to 454 technology, SOLiD library DNA fragments are ligated to oligonucleotide adapters, attached to beads, and clonally amplified by emulsion PCR. Then, beads are immobilized onto a derivatized-glass flow-cell surface, and sequencing begins by annealing a primer oligonucleotide complementary to the adapter at the adapter–template junction (Voelkerding et al. 2009). The primer is oriented to provide a 5′ phosphate group for ligation to interrogation probes during the first "ligation sequencing" step. The 8-mer interrogation probe consists of (in the 3′-to-5′ direction) two probe-specific bases followed by six degenerate bases with one of four fluorescent dyes at the 5′ end. The two probe-specific bases consist of one of 16 possible two-base combinations. For the first ligation sequencing step, the 16 possible two-base interrogation combinations, and a thermostable ligase are present. There is a probe competition for template sequence annealing located adjacent to the primer. Post-annealing, ligation occurs and a wash to remove unbound probe follows (Mardis 2008). The fluorescent signal is recorded before cleavage of the ligated probes, a wash is performed to remove the fluor, and the 5′ phosphate group is regenerated. In the next steps, ligation of interrogation probes to the 5′ phosphate group of the preceding 5-mer is performed. The first primer is extended by seven cycles of ligation, known as a round. Denaturation of the synthesized strand is performed and a new sequencing primer offset by one base in the adapter sequence (n1) is annealed. A total of five rounds are performed, each with a new successively offset primer, permitting each nucleotide to be sequenced twice. The sequence can be obtained by examining the 16 two-base possible interrogation probes.

At the end of 2007, ABI released the first SOLiD system with a read length of 35 bp and an output of 3 Gb per run. Capping, to decrease signal deterioration, coupled with high-fidelity ligation chemistry and interrogation of each nucleotide base twice during independent ligation cycles yields SOLiD can reach an accuracy of 99.9 % for a known target at a 15-fold sequence coverage over sequence reads of 25 nucleotides (Liu et al. 2012). Five system upgrades followed in the next 3 years. In 2010, the SOLiD 5500xl sequencing system was released with improvements that included improved read length, accuracy, and data output of 85 bp, 99.99 %, and 30 Gb per run, respectively. The shortcoming of this platform is the short-read length. The applications of this platform include whole-genome resequencing, targeted resequencing, transcriptome profiling, and epigenome. Like other NGS systems, SOLiD's computational infrastructure is expensive. A complete run is 7 days and produces about 4 TB of raw data. Automation can be used in library preparations via a Tecan system which integrated a Covaris A and Roche 454 REM e system.

2.6   Benchtop Sequencers

Ion Personal Genome Machine (PGM) and MiSeq were launched by Ion Torrent and Illumina (Fig. 1.1). They are both small in size and feature fast turnover rates but limited data throughput. They are suitable for clinical applications and small laboratories.

2.6.1   Personal Genome Machine (PGM)

In 2010, Ion Torrent released the Ion PGM which is based on semiconductor sequencing technology (Fig. 1.1). A proton is released when nucleotide incorporation, by a polymerase, extends a DNA molecule based on complementation. Nucleotide addition or lack of is detected in the PGM by measuring the pH difference. Specifically, no voltage difference is detected when a nucleotide is added to the chip. However, the voltage will double if two appropriate nucleotides are added (Flusberg et al. 2010).

The PGM is the first commercial sequencing machine that does not utilize fluorescence signal detection to obtain sequence information. Consequently, the platform permits higher speed, lower cost, and smaller instrument size. For example, it can process 200 bp reads in 2 h with sample preparation time that is less than 6 h. The sequence quality of PGM is more stable, compared to the decreasing quality of the HiSeq 2000 after 50 cycles, as explained by fluorescent signal decay. It was shown that PGM has a stable quality along sequencing reads and a good performance on mismatch accuracies, but has rather a bias in detection of indels (Liu et al. 2012). Moreover, the GC depth distribution is better in PGM when compared to the HiSeq 2000. Ion Torrent has already released Ion 314 and 316, and 318 chips. The chips are different in the number of wells resulting in higher production within the same sequencing time. The Ion 318 v2 chip enables the production of greater than 1.2–2 Gb data in 2 h with a read length of 400 bp.

2.6.2   Illumina's MiSeq

In 2011, MiSeq, a benchtop sequencer, was launched with shared sequencing technology with HiSeq 2000 (Fig. 1.1). Its latest output generates 8.5 Gb per run (2×250 bp paired-end reads) in about 39 h. At the end of 2013 it will produce 15 Gb per run in about 48 h with a length of 300 bp. A compact, all-in-one platform incorporates cluster generation, paired-end fluidics, sequencing by synthesis chemistry, and complete data analysis. An intuitive touch screen interface makes for simple instrument operation. Plug-and-play reagents with RFID tracking make for added convenience. MiSeq eliminates the need for auxiliary hardware and computing resources, saving valuable laboratory bench space. This system allows assembly of small genomes or targeted gene panels with unmatched accuracy, especially within homopolymer regions. It uses the shortest sample-to-data workflow among all benchtop sequencers.

2.7   NGS Analysis Strategies

After obtaining the sequence data from the sequencing, NGS reads (short DNA fragments) are aligned with the reference genome to find the genetic variations (Ruffalo et al. 2011). For bioinformaticians with the Linux system experience, there are numerous open source aligners. A summary about the sources for downloading various software packages is given at (http://en.wikipedia.org/wiki/List_of_sequence_alignment_software). In contrast, one stop commercial solutions for data analysis have emerged (Softgenetics NextGENe) and some of them are web-based cloud computational servers (e.g., www.dnanexus.com). The depth of coverage can be defined as the number of times each nucleotide is independently sequenced in different reads (Bao et al. 2011). Generally, a large number of variant differences between an individual's sequence and a reference sequence is expected to be obtained after the NGS analysis is complete.

The next step of the analysis process aims at distinguishing the potential disease causative variants from the benign SNPs by using a combined filtering approach based on mutation type, previously identified mutations, predictions of pathogenicity, knowledge database searches, inheritance patterns, and phenotype consideration (a detailed description is in Chap. 8). Generally, assumptions are made to identify pathogenic mutations using NGS data. Mutations are assumed to have a higher penetrance and mutations that are directly affecting protein structure will have functional consequences that can be easily observed. Thus, mutation candidates are nonsynonymous mutations, insertions/deletions, and splice-site mutations. In addition, common SNPs, found in healthy individuals, are filtered out of the analysis variant set. To aid in the mutation identification, a number of databases and software packages are used to determine the meaning of variants discovered by NGS (Bao et al. 2011). The Human Gene Mutation Database (HGMD; http://www.hgmd.cf.ac.uk/ac/index.php) and dbSNP (http://www.ncbi.nlm.nih.gov/projects/SNP/) are queried to determine if the variants have previously been detected or reported in the literature for a particular disease. SIFT (http://sift.jcvi.org/) and polyPhen (http://genetics.bwh.harvard.edu/pph2/) are typically used to predict if a coding region change will have a deleterious effect on protein structure and function. Due to the complexity and amount of biological information, there are a number of knowledge-based databases that aid in the interpretation of NGS variants, namely, Online Mendelian

Inheritance in Man (OMIM; http://www.ncbi.nlm.nih.gov/omim), Kyoto Encyclopedia of Genes and Genomes (http://www.genome.jp/kegg/), and Ingenuity System Pathway Analysis (http://www.ingenuity.com/products/ipa). In addition to pathogenicity predictions, filtering by using phenotype databases in consideration of the patient's clinical features (OMIM) and patterns of inheritance among family members are usually required to identify candidates of deleterious mutations (1000 Genomes Project Consortium et al. 2010). However, designation of pathogenicity to variants is still a challenging task.

2.8   Common Sources of Errors in NGS Data

The presence of systematic false positive and negative variation troubles NGS data. Specifically, incorrect genome mapping, equipment sequencing errors, or sequencing calls of DNA fragments near the ends are responsible for false positives variants (Lin et al. 2012). For example, pyrosequencing NGS systems have systematic errors at 5–6 nucleotide homopolymer stretches (Margulies et al. 2005). To improve the accuracy, such error can be removed from the final list of variants. Furthermore, software alignment artifacts may be reduced by cross software alignment comparisons. In contrast, depth of coverage, poor capture efficiency, and difficulty in unambiguously aligning repetitive regions usually cause false negative variants (Nothnagel et al. 2011). This NGS error can be reduced by raising the threshold of the sequencing coverage to reach clinical standard accuracy such as that of Sanger sequencing (Koboldt et al. 2010). Additionally, increasing coverage reduces the error rate, specifically, for heterozygous variants. Moreover, false positive variants can be further reduced by using longer reads which consequently decreases mapping ambiguity. When longer reads are used, it is advisable to trim the end nucleotides since they have higher error rates (Ledergerber and Dessimoz 2011). Paired-end sequencing permits alignment software to find the correct target region and to reduce the interference from pseudogene regions (Nielsen et al. 2011). However, for NGS clinical sequencing panels Sanger sequencing is usually required before the final report can be issued.

2.9   Clinical Applications of NGS

Despite its errors, NGS has been employed by the research community to identify causal genes and clinical laboratories have started to apply these technologies for the diagnosis of Mendelian disorders (detailed in Chaps. 4–8). Most Mendelian disorders are caused by exonic or splice-site mutations that alter the amino acid sequence of the affected gene. The number of known mutations in human genes underlying or associated with inherited disease exceeds 110,000 in more than 3,700 different genes (entries in OMIM). NGS has brought new ways of addressing monogenic disorders. Because of its large capacity to unbiasedly survey the exome and genome, NGS is well suited in the usage of discovering the cause of rare genetic disorders (Chap. 8). When properly executed, the WES approach may dramatically reduce the required sample number needed for a successful outcome. The use of NGS has frequently resulted in identifying disease genes with even a limited number of patient samples (Fig. 1.1; Kalay et al. 2011; Krawitz et al. 2010; Kuhlenbäumer et al. 2011; Musunuru et al. 2010; Ng et al. 2010a, b; Puente et al. 2011; Simpson et al. 2011). Novel and causative variants have recently been discovered for diverse types of diseases, including neuropathy cases (Brkanac et al. 2009), Clericuzio type poikiloderma with neutropenia (Volpi et al. 2010), familial exudative vitreoretinopathy (Nikopoulos et al. 2010), immunological disorders (Bolze et al. 2010; Byun et al. 2010), intellectual disabilities (Abou Jamra et al. 2011; Shoubridge et al. 2010), cancer predisposition (Shoubridge et al. 2010), and other abnormalities (Barak et al. 2011; Bilgüvar et al. 2010; Otto et al. 2010). Novel genes for nonsyndromic (Rehman et al. 2010; Walsh et al. 2010) and syndromic (Pierce et al. 2010; Zheng et al. 2011) hearing loss were also identified recently by the targeted NGS approach. These studies show that the targeted genomic region (Rehman et al. 2010) or whole exome NGS (Pierce et al. 2010; Walsh et al. 2010), followed by verification from nonconsanguineous families, and by functional and immunolabeling examinations, can reveal critical disease-causing genes from small pedigrees.

The success of NGS in research has already resulted in its translational uses in clinical care, and many of them are for diagnostic mutation detection of focused panels of disease genes which will be covered in Chaps. 6 and 7. In clinical practice, the Cincinnati Children's Medical Center's Molecular Genetics Laboratory (http://www.cincinnatichildrens.org/service/d/diagnostic-labs/molecular-genetics/default/) offers NGS panels for fatty acid oxidation disorders, hearing loss, and immunodeficiencies, namely, bone marrow failure syndromes, chromosome breakage disorders, dyskeratosis congenital, Fanconi anemia, and severe combined immunodeficiency. Other clinical laboratories offering clinical NGS panels include Emory Genetics Laboratory, Baylor College of Medicine, GeneDx, and Prevention Genetics. The clinical uses of NGS will only continue to grow as NGS panels expand to WES analysis and eventually WGS analysis.

2.10 Summary

Many NGS technologies have been introduced in the past 8 years. Each platform possesses its advantages and disadvantages such as throughput, accuracy, run times, price, and ease of use. Due to this large array of NGS platform options, clinical laboratories are adopting the technologies that meet their specific needs. For example, the Illumina HiSeq 2500 has been the choice for large NGS panels with fast turnaround times. In contrast, Illumina's MiSeq may provide enough coverage for smaller gene panels. The use of NGS is clinical laboratories is expanding as evidenced by the increasing number of panels and laboratories offering such services (Chaps. 5–8). This expansion will continue as clinical genetic testing moves towards exome sequencing (Chap. 8).

References

1000 Genomes Project Consortium, Abecasis GR, Altshuler D et al (2010) A map of human genome variation from population-scale sequencing. Nature 467:1061–1073. doi:10.1038/nature09534

Abou Jamra R, Philippe O, Raas-Rothschild A et al (2011) Adaptor protein complex 4 deficiency causes severe autosomal-recessive intellectual disability, progressive spastic paraplegia, shy character, and short stature. Am J Hum Genet 88:788–795. doi:10.1016/j.ajhg.2011.04.019

Bao S, Jiang R, Kwan W et al (2011) Evaluation of next-generation sequencing software in mapping and assembly. J Hum Genet 56:406–414. doi:10.1038/jhg.2011.43

Barak T, Kwan KY, Louvi A et al (2011) Recessive LAMC3 mutations cause malformations of occipital cortical development. Nat Genet 43:590–594. doi:10.1038/ng.836

Bick D, Dimmock D (2011) Whole exome and whole genome sequencing. Curr Opin Pediatr 23:594–600. doi:10.1097/MOP.0b013e32834b20ec

Bilgüvar K, Oztürk AK, Louvi A et al (2010) Whole-exome sequencing identifies recessive WDR62 mutations in severe brain malformations. Nature 467:207–210. doi:10.1038/nature09327

Bolze A, Byun M, McDonald D et al (2010) Whole-exome-sequencing-based discovery of human FADD deficiency. Am J Hum Genet 87:873–881. doi:10.1016/j.ajhg.2010.10.028

Borgström E, Lundin S, Lundeberg J (2011) Large scale library generation for high throughput sequencing. PLoS One 6:e19119. doi:10.1371/journal.pone.0019119

Brkanac Z, Spencer D, Shendure J et al (2009) IFRD1 is a candidate gene for SMNA on chromosome 7q22-q23. Am J Hum Genet 84:692–697. doi:10.1016/j.ajhg.2009.04.008

Byun M, Abhyankar A, Lelarge V et al (2010) Whole-exome sequencing-based discovery of STIM1 deficiency in a child with fatal classic Kaposi sarcoma. J Exp Med 207:2307–2312. doi:10.1084/jem.20101597

Clark MJ, Chen R, Lam HYK et al (2011) Performance comparison of exome DNA sequencing technologies. Nat Biotechnol 29:908–914. doi:10.1038/nbt.1975

Eid J, Fehr A, Gray J et al (2009) Real-time DNA sequencing from single polymerase molecules. Science 323:133–138. doi:10.1126/science.1162986

Flusberg BA, Webster DR, Lee JH et al (2010) Direct detection of DNA methylation during single-molecule, real-time sequencing. Nat Methods 7:461–465. doi:10.1038/nmeth.1459

Huse SM, Huber JA, Morrison HG et al (2007) Accuracy and quality of massively parallel DNA pyrosequencing. Genome Biol 8:R143. doi:10.1186/gb-2007-8-7-r143

Kalay E, Yigit G, Aslan Y et al (2011) CEP152 is a genome maintenance protein disrupted in Seckel syndrome. Nat Genet 43:23–26. doi:10.1038/ng.725

Koboldt DC, Ding L, Mardis ER, Wilson RK (2010) Challenges of sequencing human genomes. Brief Bioinform 11:484–498. doi:10.1093/bib/bbq016

Krawitz PM, Schweiger MR, Rödelsperger C et al (2010) Identity-by-descent filtering of exome sequence data identifies PIGV mutations in hyperphosphatasia mental retardation syndrome. Nat Genet 42:827–829. doi:10.1038/ng.653

Kuhlenbäumer G, Hullmann J, Appenzeller S (2011) Novel genomic techniques open new avenues in the analysis of monogenic disorders. Hum Mutat 32:144–151. doi:10.1002/humu.21400

Ledergerber C, Dessimoz C (2011) Base-calling for next-generation sequencing platforms. Brief Bioinform 12:489–497. doi:10.1093/bib/bbq077

Lin X, Tang W, Ahmad S et al (2012) Applications of targeted gene capture and next-generation sequencing technologies in studies of human deafness and other genetic disabilities. Hear Res 288:67–76. doi:10.1016/j.heares.2012.01.004

Liu L, Li Y, Li S et al (2012) Comparison of next-generation sequencing systems. J Biomed Biotechnol 2012:251364. doi:10.1155/2012/251364

Mardis ER (2008) The impact of next-generation sequencing technology on genetics. Trends Genet 24:133–141. doi:10.1016/j.tig.2007.12.007

Margulies M, Egholm M, Altman WE et al (2005) Genome sequencing in microfabricated high-density picolitre reactors. Nature 437:376–380. doi:10.1038/nature03959

Maxam AM, Gilbert W (1977) A new method for sequencing DNA. Proc Natl Acad Sci U S A 74:560–564

Musunuru K, Pirruccello JP, Do R et al (2010) Exome sequencing, ANGPTL3 mutations, and familial combined hypolipidemia. N Engl J Med 363:2220–2227. doi:10.1056/NEJMoa1002926

Ng SB, Bigham AW, Buckingham KJ et al (2010a) Exome sequencing identifies MLL2 mutations as a cause of Kabuki syndrome. Nat Genet 42:790–793. doi:10.1038/ng.646

Ng SB, Buckingham KJ, Lee C et al (2010b) Exome sequencing identifies the cause of a mendelian disorder. Nat Genet 42:30–35. doi:10.1038/ng.499

Nielsen R, Paul JS, Albrechtsen A, Song YS (2011) Genotype and SNP calling from next-generation sequencing data. Nat Rev Genet 12:443–451. doi:10.1038/nrg2986

Nikopoulos K, Gilissen C, Hoischen A et al (2010) Next-generation sequencing of a 40 Mb linkage interval reveals TSPAN12 mutations in patients with familial exudative vitreoretinopathy. Am J Hum Genet 86:240–247. doi:10.1016/j.ajhg.2009.12.016

Nothnagel M, Herrmann A, Wolf A et al (2011) Technology-specific error signatures in the 1000 Genomes Project data. Hum Genet 130:505–516. doi:10.1007/s00439-011-0971-3

Otto EA, Hurd TW, Airik R et al (2010) Candidate exome capture identifies mutation of SDCCAG8 as the cause of a retinal-renal ciliopathy. Nat Genet 42:840–850. doi:10.1038/ng.662

Pierce SB, Walsh T, Chisholm KM et al (2010) Mutations in the DBP-deficiency protein HSD17B4 cause ovarian dysgenesis, hearing loss, and ataxia of Perrault Syndrome. Am J Hum Genet 87:282–288. doi:10.1016/j.ajhg.2010.07.007

Puente XS, Quesada V, Osorio FG et al (2011) Exome sequencing and functional analysis identifies BANF1 mutation as the cause of a hereditary progeroid syndrome. Am J Hum Genet 88:650–656. doi:10.1016/j.ajhg.2011.04.010

Rehman AU, Morell RJ, Belyantseva IA et al (2010) Targeted capture and next-generation sequencing identifies C9orf75, encoding taperin, as the mutated gene in nonsyndromic deafness DFNB79. Am J Hum Genet 86:378–388. doi:10.1016/j.ajhg.2010.01.030

Rothberg JM, Hinz W, Rearick TM et al (2011) An integrated semiconductor device enabling non-optical genome sequencing. Nature 475:348–352. doi:10.1038/nature10242

Ruffalo M, LaFramboise T, Koyutürk M (2011) Comparative analysis of algorithms for next-generation sequencing read alignment. Bioinformatics (Oxf Engl) 27:2790–2796. doi:10.1093/bioinformatics/btr477

Ruparel H, Bi L, Li Z et al (2005) Design and synthesis of a 3'-O-allyl photocleavable fluorescent nucleotide as a reversible terminator for DNA sequencing by synthesis. Proc Natl Acad Sci U S A 102:5932–5937. doi:10.1073/pnas.0501962102

Sanger F, Nicklen S, Coulson AR (1977) DNA sequencing with chain-terminating inhibitors. Proc Natl Acad Sci U S A 74:5463–5467

Shendure J, Porreca GJ, Reppas NB et al (2005) Accurate multiplex polony sequencing of an evolved bacterial genome. Science 309:1728–1732. doi:10.1126/science.1117389

Shoubridge C, Tarpey PS, Abidi F et al (2010) Mutations in the guanine nucleotide exchange factor gene IQSEC2 cause nonsyndromic intellectual disability. Nat Genet 42:486–488. doi:10.1038/ng.588

Simpson MA, Irving MD, Asilmaz E et al (2011) Mutations in NOTCH2 cause Hajdu-Cheney syndrome, a disorder of severe and progressive bone loss. Nat Genet 43:303–305. doi:10.1038/ng.779

Voelkerding KV, Dames SA, Durtschi JD (2009) Next-generation sequencing: from basic research to diagnostics. Clin Chem 55:641–658. doi:10.1373/clinchem.2008.112789

Volpi L, Roversi G, Colombo EA et al (2010) Targeted next-generation sequencing appoints c16orf57 as clericuzio-type poikiloderma with neutropenia gene. Am J Hum Genet 86:72–76. doi:10.1016/j.ajhg.2009.11.014

Walsh T, Shahin H, Elkan-Miller T et al (2010) Whole exome sequencing and homozygosity mapping identify mutation in the cell polarity protein GPSM2 as the cause of nonsyndromic hearing loss DFNB82. Am J Hum Genet 87:90–94. doi:10.1016/j.ajhg.2010.05.010

Wheeler DA, Srinivasan M, Egholm M et al (2008) The complete genome of an individual by massively parallel DNA sequencing. Nature 452:872–876. doi:10.1038/nature06884

Zheng J, Miller KK, Yang T et al (2011) Carcinoembryonic antigen-related cell adhesion molecule 16 interacts with alpha-tectorin and is mutated in autosomal dominant hearing loss (DFNA4). Proc Natl Acad Sci U S A 108:4218–4223. doi:10.1073/pnas.1005842108

Chapter 3
A Review of DNA Enrichment Technologies

3.1 Introduction

Next-generation–sequencing (NGS) technologies, by sequencing hundreds of thousands to millions of DNA templates in parallel, resulted in higher throughput (Gb scale) and lowered sequencing cost (Mardis 2008; Shendure and Ji 2008). This has permitted the definition of the entire genome as well as the differences that exist between them. The ultimate goal is to routinely perform whole-genome sequencing to allow us to gain a deeper understanding of genetic variation and to define its role in phenotypic variation and the pathogenesis of complex traits (Mamanova et al. 2010). Due to the cost and time limitations, it is not yet feasible to sequence large numbers of complex genomes. Therefore, a significant effort has focused on the development of "target enrichment" methods, in which genomic regions are selectively captured from a DNA sample before sequencing (Fig. 3.1). This approach is more time- and cost-effective, and the resulting data are considerably less cumbersome to analyze, except in the case of exome capture (Chap. 8). Several approaches to target enrichment have been developed, and the performance parameters vary from one to another: (1) sensitivity, or the percentage of the target bases that are represented by one or more sequence reads; (2) specificity, or the percentage of sequences that map to the intended targets; (3) uniformity, or the variability in sequence coverage across target regions; (4) reproducibility, or how closely results obtained from replicate experiments correlate; (5) cost; (6) ease of use; and (7) amount of DNA required per experiment, or per megabase of target (Mamanova et al. 2010).

To enrich for regions of interest that range in size from hundreds of kb to the whole exome, genomic enrichment steps, both traditional and novel, are being incorporated into overall experimental designs (Voelkerding et al. 2009). Traditional overlapping long-range PCR amplicons (approximately 5–10 kb) can only be used for up to several hundred kb. More recently, enrichment based on hybridization of fragmented genomic DNA to oligonucleotide capture probes has been successfully achieved by several groups (Albert et al. 2007; Hodges et al. 2007; Okou et al. 2007;

C.A. Valencia et al., *Next Generation Sequencing Technologies in Medical Genetics*,
SpringerBriefs in Genetics, DOI 10.1007/978-1-4614-9032-6_3,
© C. Alexander Valencia 2013

a Molecular inversion probes - yields 10,000 exons

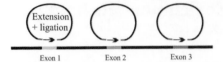

b Droplet PCR amplification- yields up to 4000 amplicons

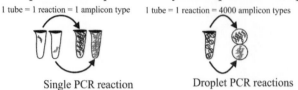

c Hybridization-based capture - captures > 10,000 exons, up to exome

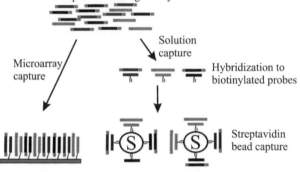

Fig. 3.1 Target enrichment methods. (**a**) In molecular inversion probes (MIPs), probes composed of a universal spacer region flanked by target-specific sequences are designed for each amplicon. The gap is filled by a DNA polymerase and a ligase following probe annealing to the target region. The target DNA is PCR-amplified after genomic digestion and sequenced. (**b**) In a typical PCR, a single amplicon is generated by one reaction. By RDT, up to 4,000 primer pairs are used simultaneously in a single reaction. (**c**) By hybridization-based captures, genomic DNA libraries containing adaptors are hybridized to target-specific probes either on a microarray surface or in solution. The target DNA is eluted and sequenced after removal of background DNA by washing (adapted from Mamanova et al. 2010)

Porreca et al. 2007). Capture probes can be immobilized on a solid surface (Roche NimbleGen, Agilent Technologies, and Febit) or used in solution (Agilent). Another enrichment approach that relies on the use of molecular inversion probes (MIPs) was initially developed for multiplex target detection and SNP genotyping (Ding et al. 2008; Kim et al. 2008). In principle, single-stranded oligonucleotides, consisting of a common linker flanked by target-specific sequences, anneal to their target sequence and become circularized by a ligase (Hodges et al. 2007). In an alternative enrichment approach, developed by RainDance Technologies (RDT), individual pairs of PCR primers for the genomic regions of interest are segregated in water in emulsion droplets and then pooled to create a primer library (Tewhey et al. 2009). Separately, emulsion droplets containing genomic DNA and PCR reagents are prepared. Following the merging of the droplets, DNA is amplified by the PCR and subsequently processed for NGS.

The intent of this chapter is to provide a cursory view of the enrichment technologies that are commercially available, to lay the principles of each technology, and provide examples of which methods have been used in clinical laboratories.

3.2   Non-hybridization-Based Enrichment Methods

3.2.1   Molecular Inversion Probes

PCR-based non-hybridization gene enrichment schemes include MIPs (Fig. 3.1; Deng et al. 2009; Porreca et al. 2007; Turner et al. 2009). Briefly, single-stranded oligonucleotides with a common linker flanked by target-specific sequences are annealed to their target sequence and a ligase circularizes them (Landegren et al. 2004; Nilsson et al. 1994). Any uncircularized molecule is digested by exonuclease treatment to reduce background, and circularized molecules are PCR-amplified via primers directed at the common linker. To perform exon capture in combination with NGS, a DNA polymerase can be used to gap-fill between target-specific MIP sequences designed to flank a full or partial exon, before ligase-driven circularization, thus capturing a copy of the intervening sequence (Porreca et al. 2007). The assay is afflicted by low uniformity due to inefficiencies of the capture reaction. However, an optimized, simplified protocol for MIP-based exon capture has been reported (Turner et al. 2009). The main disadvantages of using MIPs for target enrichment are capture uniformity compared to hybridization-based methods. Additionally, MIP oligonucleotides are costly and not readily available in large numbers to cover large target sets. In contrast, the current view of MIP-based capture followed by direct sequencing may be most relevant for projects involving relatively small numbers of targets but large numbers of samples. Unfortunately, this method was never developed into a commercially available product.

3.2.2   Highly Multiplex Droplet PCR

For over 20 years, PCR has been the method of choice for amplification before sequencing a sample (Mamanova et al. 2010). This approach is compatible with Sanger sequencing because a single amplicon is generated that can be easily subsequently sequenced and the length of an amplicon is comparable to the length of sequence produced. PCR may be compatible with NGS platforms as long as a large number of PCR products for a region of interest can be generated. However, failure to amplify a high percentage of regions is the limitation of highly multiplexed PCR. Moreover, multiplexes are difficult to decipher as to which PCR products are amplifying and which one are not unless sequencing verification is performed. The parallel use of many primer pairs can generate a high level of nonspecific amplification, caused by interaction between the primers.

To overcome these shortcomings, PCR amplification, by RDT, in a microfluidic environment has been successfully performed (Tewhey et al. 2009). In essence, oil microdroplets segregate thousands of individual PCRs in the same reaction tube (Fig. 3.1). Specifically, each droplet supports an independent PCR by containing a single primer pair with genomic DNA and other reagents. The droplet population is hundreds to thousands of distinct primer pairs and is subjected to thermal cycling, after which this emulsion is broken and products are recovered. The mixture of DNA amplicons are subjected to shotgun library construction and NGS sequencing. This technology prevents different primer pairs from interacting with each other and removes the key constraint of multiplex PCR. However, the initial cost of purchasing a large amount of PCR primers and the cost of equipment are very substantial in commercial offerings. This technology has been recently applied in clinical laboratories to aid in the diagnosis of congenital disorders of glycosylation, congenital muscular dystrophy, and hearing loss (Jones et al. 2011; Sivakumaran et al. 2013; Valencia et al. 2012, 2013). The application of this technology to congenital muscular dystrophy and hearing loss is discussed in detail in Chaps. 6 and 7.

3.3   Hybridization-Based Enrichment Methods

Hybridization-based methods are the most popular targeted enrichment strategies and have been extended to capture the whole human exome reliably (Clark et al. 2011; Majewski et al. 2011). Such an approach can be classified as liquid-based hybridization (Bainbridge et al. 2010) or solid phase-based (e.g., microarray-based) hybridization (Choi et al. 2009; Hodges et al. 2007), depending on how the reactions are experimentally implemented.

3.3.1   Solid Phase Capture

The principle of enrichment through direct selection is well known and it includes several procedural steps, namely, shotgun fragment library hybridization to immobilized probe, nonspecific hybrids are washed away, and captured DNA is eluted (Lovett et al. 1991). Roche NimbleGen made this technology compatible with NGS (Fig. 3.1; Albert et al. 2007; Hodges et al. 2009; Okou et al. 2007). Such a method can usually enrich targets by about 1,000- to 2,000-fold in one round of hybridization reaction (Albert et al. 2007). The enrichment efficiency has been increased by multiple enrichment cycles (Summerer et al. 2009). Originally, a single microarray with 385,000 probes was hybridized to a library DNA (HD1 NimbleGen array) with a region of interest around 4–5 Mb. More recent microarrays contain 2.1 million probes and can capture greater than 60 Mb, the exome. Following the capture, NGS can be performed using any of the sequencing platforms including Illumina HiSeq 2500. In contrast, Agilent's Capture Arrays, with only 244,000 probes, are the most direct competitor to NimbleGen's HD1 arrays. One key factor for a successful target enrichment outcome is the probe design, which is dependent on gene annotation databases such as the RefSeq database. Therefore, unknown disease causing genes, noncoding genomic regions, and regulatory sequences are not included in the designs. Also high GC percentage regions are poorly captured (Okou et al. 2007).

Microarray target enrichment of large genomic regions is faster and less labor-intensive than comparable PCR-based approaches. However, the drawbacks of this technology are that the hardware is expensive and the DNA requirement is large, around 10–15 μg, though this is irrespective of whether the capture experiment is for 100 kb or an entire exome (Mamanova et al. 2010). In addition, the number of microarrays that can be processed by a single person per day is a limiting factor to scale up the operation in a clinical laboratory. Despite its disadvantages, solid phase hybridization methods have successfully been used for enrichment of genes involved in deafness, retinitis pigmentosa, cardiomyopathies, and immunodeficiencies (Daiger et al. 2010; Ghosh et al. 2012; Meder et al. 2011; Shearer et al. 2010; Simpson et al. 2011).

3.3.2 Solution-Based Capture

Both Agilent and NimbleGen have developed and commercialized solution captures. Experimentally, the capture consists of a number of general steps. Biotinylated DNA or RNA probes are hybridized, for several days, with fragmented target DNA. The DNA/probe hybrids in the solution are captured by magnetic streptavidin beads immobilized by a strong magnet. DNA fragments not targeted in the liquid phase are removed by repeated washes. Targeted DNA fragments are eluted from the beads by increasing the pH with NaOH in order to break the biotin streptavidin bond and degrade the RNA probes. Only the enriched DNA fragments are sequenced by NGS protocols.

Solution captures were introduced to overcome the aforementioned disadvantages of microarray captures (Fig. 3.1). Agilent (150-mer RNA probes) and NimbleGen (60- to 90-mer DNA probes) solution captures differ in regard to the nature of the probes. Solution target enrichment can be performed in 96-well plates, using a thermal cycler, so it is more readily scalable than microarray enrichment and does not require expensive equipment (Mamanova et al. 2010). Microarray and solution captures use specific probes designed to target regions of interest. The distinguishing feature is the probe to library ratio during the hybridization. Microarray target enrichment uses a vast excess of DNA library over probes, whereas, solution capture has an excess of probes over template, driving the hybridization reaction further to completion using a smaller quantity of initial library (Gnirke et al. 2009). In terms of performance, for smaller target sizes (~3.5 Mb), the uniformity and specificity of sequences obtained from a solution capture experiment tend to be slightly higher than those of microarray capture (Mamanova et al. 2010). In contrast, for whole-exome captures, the NimbleGen platform, which is the only one to use high-density overlapping baits, covers fewer genomic regions than the other platform but requires the least amount of sequencing to sensitively detect small variants (Clark et al. 2011). Agilent is able to detect a greater total number of variants with additional sequencing. Importantly, it was shown that that exome sequencing can detect additional small variants missed by WGS (Clark et al. 2011). Significantly, solution captures have been used for mutation detection in congenital muscular dystrophy and hearing loss (Shearer et al. 2010; Valencia et al. 2012).

3.4   Summary

Advances in enrichment technologies, alongside NGS platforms, are accelerating the discovery of genetic disorders at a rapid pace and are beginning to make their way into clinical practice. Focused panel and exome NGS data are now being generated by clinical laboratories at major genome centers nationwide by employing enrichment technologies. The choice of specific enrichment method depends on the sample number, the target size, and performance. For example, RDT has been the method of choice for small (<1 Mb) NGS panels, but hybridization methods are routinely used for exome capture. Interpreting the data with the aim of identifying pathogenic mutations, among thousands to millions of variants, is still challenging and the creation of clinical databases containing NGS results from a large number of normal controls will greatly aid in the process. In the near future, NGS data may help define genetic profiles of patients and will be a step towards personalized medical care.

References

Albert TJ, Molla MN, Muzny DM et al (2007) Direct selection of human genomic loci by microarray hybridization. Nat Methods 4:903–905. doi:10.1038/nmeth1111

Bainbridge MN, Wang M, Burgess DL et al (2010) Whole exome capture in solution with 3 Gbp of data. Genome Biol 11:R62. doi:10.1186/gb-2010-11-6-r62

Choi M, Scholl UI, Ji W et al (2009) Genetic diagnosis by whole exome capture and massively parallel DNA sequencing. Proc Natl Acad Sci U S A 106:19096–19101. doi:10.1073/pnas.0910672106

Clark MJ, Chen R, Lam HYK et al (2011) Performance comparison of exome DNA sequencing technologies. Nat Biotechnol 29:908–914. doi:10.1038/nbt.1975

Daiger SP, Sullivan LS, Bowne SJ et al (2010) Targeted high-throughput DNA sequencing for gene discovery in retinitis pigmentosa. Adv Exp Med Biol 664:325–331. doi:10.1007/978-1-4419-1399-9_37

Deng J, Shoemaker R, Xie B et al (2009) Targeted bisulfite sequencing reveals changes in DNA methylation associated with nuclear reprogramming. Nat Biotechnol 27:353–360. doi:10.1038/nbt.1530

Ding L, Getz G, Wheeler DA et al (2008) Somatic mutations affect key pathways in lung adenocarcinoma. Nature 455:1069–1075. doi:10.1038/nature07423

Ghosh S, Krux F, Binder V et al (2012) Array-based sequence capture and next-generation sequencing for the identification of primary immunodeficiencies. Scand J Immunol 75:350–354. doi:10.1111/j.1365-3083.2011.02658.x

Gnirke A, Melnikov A, Maguire J et al (2009) Solution hybrid selection with ultra-long oligonucleotides for massively parallel targeted sequencing. Nat Biotechnol 27:182–189. doi:10.1038/nbt.1523

Hodges E, Xuan Z, Balija V et al (2007) Genome-wide in situ exon capture for selective resequencing. Nat Genet 39:1522–1527. doi:10.1038/ng.2007.42

Hodges E, Rooks M, Xuan Z et al (2009) Hybrid selection of discrete genomic intervals on custom-designed microarrays for massively parallel sequencing. Nat Protoc 4:960–974. doi:10.1038/nprot.2009.68

Jones MA, Bhide S, Chin E et al (2011) Targeted polymerase chain reaction-based enrichment and next-generation sequencing for diagnostic testing of congenital disorders of glycosylation. Genet Med 13:921–932. doi:10.1097/GIM.0b013e318226fbf2

Kim PM, Lam HYK, Urban AE et al (2008) Analysis of copy number variants and segmental duplications in the human genome: evidence for a change in the process of formation in recent evolutionary history. Genome Res 18:1865–1874. doi:10.1101/gr.081422.108

Landegren U, Schallmeiner E, Nilsson M et al (2004) Molecular tools for a molecular medicine: analyzing genes, transcripts and proteins using padlock and proximity probes. J Mol Recognit 17:194–197. doi:10.1002/jmr.664

Lovett M, Kere J, Hinton LM (1991) Direct selection: a method for the isolation of cDNAs encoded by large genomic regions. Proc Natl Acad Sci U S A 88:9628–9632

Majewski J, Schwartzentruber J, Lalonde E et al (2011) What can exome sequencing do for you? J Med Genet 48:580–589. doi:10.1136/jmedgenet-2011-100223

Mamanova L, Coffey AJ, Scott CE et al (2010) Target-enrichment strategies for next-generation sequencing. Nat Methods 7:111–118. doi:10.1038/nmeth.1419

Mardis ER (2008) The impact of next-generation sequencing technology on genetics. Trends Genet 24:133–141. doi:10.1016/j.tig.2007.12.007

Meder B, Haas J, Keller A et al (2011) Targeted next-generation sequencing for the molecular genetic diagnostics of cardiomyopathies. Circ Cardiovasc Genet 4:110–122. doi:10.1161/CIRCGENETICS.110.958322

Nilsson M, Malmgren H, Samiotaki M et al (1994) Padlock probes: circularizing oligonucleotides for localized DNA detection. Science 265:2085–2088

Okou DT, Steinberg KM, Middle C et al (2007) Microarray-based genomic selection for high-throughput resequencing. Nat Methods 4:907–909. doi:10.1038/nmeth1109

Porreca GJ, Zhang K, Li JB et al (2007) Multiplex amplification of large sets of human exons. Nat Methods 4:931–936. doi:10.1038/nmeth1110

Shearer AE, DeLuca AP, Hildebrand MS et al (2010) Comprehensive genetic testing for hereditary hearing loss using massively parallel sequencing. Proc Natl Acad Sci U S A 107:21104–21109. doi:10.1073/pnas.1012989107

Shendure J, Ji H (2008) Next-generation DNA sequencing. Nat Biotechnol 26:1135–1145. doi:10.1038/nbt1486

Simpson DA, Clark GR, Alexander S et al (2011) Molecular diagnosis for heterogeneous genetic diseases with targeted high-throughput DNA sequencing applied to retinitis pigmentosa. J Med Genet 48:145–151. doi:10.1136/jmg.2010.083568

Sivakumaran TA, Husami A, Kissell D et al (2013) Performance evaluation of the next-generation sequencing approach for molecular diagnosis of hereditary hearing loss. Otolaryngol Head Neck Surg 148:1007–1016. doi:10.1177/0194599813482294

Summerer D, Wu H, Haase B et al (2009) Microarray-based multicycle-enrichment of genomic subsets for targeted next-generation sequencing. Genome Res 19:1616–1621. doi:10.1101/gr.091942.109

Tewhey R, Warner JB, Nakano M et al (2009) Microdroplet-based PCR enrichment for large-scale targeted sequencing. Nat Biotechnol 27:1025–1031. doi:10.1038/nbt.1583

Turner EH, Lee C, Ng SB et al (2009) Massively parallel exon capture and library-free resequencing across 16 genomes. Nat Methods 6:315–316. doi:10.1038/nmeth.f.248

Valencia CA, Rhodenizer D, Bhide S et al (2012) Assessment of target enrichment platforms using massively parallel sequencing for the mutation detection for congenital muscular dystrophy. J Mol Diagn 14:233–246. doi:10.1016/j.jmoldx.2012.01.009

Valencia CA, Ankala A, Rhodenizer D et al (2013) Comprehensive mutation analysis for congenital muscular dystrophy: a clinical PCR-based enrichment and next-generation sequencing panel. PLoS One 8:e53083. doi:10.1371/journal.pone.0053083

Voelkerding KV, Dames SA, Durtschi JD (2009) Next-generation sequencing: from basic research to diagnostics. Clin Chem 55:641–658. doi:10.1373/clinchem.2008.112789

Part II
Clinical Applications of
Next-Generation–Sequencing

Chapter 4
Application of Next-Generation–Sequencing to the Diagnosis of Genetic Disorders: A Brief Overview

4.1 Introduction

Next-generation–sequencing (NGS) holds a number of advantages over traditional Sanger sequencing, the most obvious being able to do panel testing in a shorter span of time at a lower cost (Hu et al. 2009). A number of phenotypically similar diseases can have a number of different genetic causes (Hoischen et al. 2010). This genetic heterogeneity, seen in congenital muscular dystrophies (Chap. 6), congenital disorders of glycosylation (CDG), and hearing loss (Chap. 7), can be addressed by NGS by simply sequencing all genes related to specific phenotypes (Rehman et al. 2010; Lim et al. 2011; Valencia et al. 2012). In the case of CDG, NGS is a time- and cost-effective tool for comprehensive mutations screening of metabolic diseases caused by mutations in different genes of a common pathway. In addition, its use can be applied to disorders that have a variable presentation but can raise flags for a certain set of diseases such as mitochondrial defects. One distinct advantage can be seen in the field of cancer genetics where panel testing can save a significant amount of time by reaching a diagnosis (Chan et al. 2012). An interesting application of NGS is in the application of noninvasive prenatal diagnosis of aneuploidies and trisomies 21, 18, and 13 (Chap. 5; Chiu et al. 2008).

In this chapter, we discuss the recent application of NGS in the diagnosis of a number of genetic disorders. We briefly introduce each genetic disorder and mention the corresponding gene panel that has been examined via NGS technologies to address the issue of genetic heterogeneity. We begin by introducing CDG in the next section to demonstrate how NGS can be used to screen for mutations in different genes of a common metabolic pathway.

C.A. Valencia et al., *Next Generation Sequencing Technologies in Medical Genetics*, SpringerBriefs in Genetics, DOI 10.1007/978-1-4614-9032-6_4, © C. Alexander Valencia 2013

4.2   Congenital Disorders of Glycosylation

CDG are a group of disorders, which have a variable presentation including dys-morphic features, developmental delay, ataxia, seizures, liver fibrosis, retinopathy, cardiac dysfunction, and coagulopathies (Jones et al. 2011). About 50 % of proteins in the body are N-glycosylated, which is reflected in the clinical presentation of these disorders. There is major overlap with other disorders in terms of presentation which increases the chance of them being missed during the diagnostic work-up. Their estimated prevalence is about 1 in 20,000; however, this may be higher as these disorders are underdiagnosed.

Patients are classified as having either type 1 or 2 disorder based on the pattern of serum transferrin on electrophoresis. This is, however, a screening test and car-ries a high rate of false positives and negatives. In addition, a number of disorders may be missed, as they do not have abnormal transferrin. Approximately, greater than 30 different types of CDG have been described to be caused by defects in dif-ferent gene products. Additional methodologies include using HPLC techniques to evaluate linked oligosaccharide levels as well as analysis of the glycan structure by MALDI-TOF-MS. An initial biochemical diagnosis may lead to clear diagnosis and subsequent relevant Sanger sequencing of the gene; however, in about 40 % of cases this might not be the case. It is here that NGS panel testing can offer a tremendous advantage over the gold standard of Sanger sequencing.

Jones et al. reported the validation studies of an NGS CDG panel using 12 blinded positive control samples (Jones et al. 2011). Technically, both RainDance and Fluidigm platforms were used for sequence enrichment and targeted amplifica-tion and the SOLiD platform was the sequencer of choice. The disease-causing mutations were identified by NGS for all 12 positive controls. Moreover, they pro-pose an algorithmic process to improve the diagnosis, based on a combination of biochemical and molecular tests. If clear diagnosis can be established based on clinical features and biochemical profile, Sanger sequencing for the relevant gene should be performed. However, if clinical suspicion remains without any clear bio-chemical diagnosis, NGS panel testing should be pursued. The panel consists of 25 genes (*ALG2*, *ALG3*, *ALG6*, *ALG8*, *ALG9*, *ATP6V0A2*, *B4GALT1*, *COG1*, *COG7*, *COG8*, *DOLK*, *DPAGT1*, *DPM1*, *GNE*, *MGAT2*, *MOGS*, *MPDUI*, *MPI*, *PMM2*, *RFT1*, *SLC35A1*, *SLC35C1*, and *TUSC3*). *ALG1* was not included because it has a pseudogene and was analyzed separately as part of the panel. Potentially, two muta-tions should be identified by the panel for autosomal recessive genes and a diagno-sis reached. However, if only variants of unknown clinical significance are identified, biochemical testing, if available, needs to be performed to confirm the functional consequence of those changes. NGS offers a way to diagnose patients whose phe-notypes may not be very clear that fall under the spectrum of CDG. It offers an efficient and a relatively faster way to reach a diagnosis rather than sequentially sequencing each gene by the Sanger method.

4.3   Colon Cancer

Hereditary colon cancers are caused by a number of genes and have overlapping clinical features (Pritchard et al. 2012). Lynch syndrome, also called hereditary non-polyposis colorectal cancer, is caused by defects in mismatch repair (MMR) genes, namely, *MLH1*, *MSH2*, *MSH6*, *PMS2*, and *EPCAM*. Mutations in these genes are inherited in an autosomal dominant manner. Similarly, mutations in *APC* cause autosomal dominant familial adenomatous polyposis syndrome. Additionally, mutations in *APC* can also cause Gardner's syndrome, Turcots syndrome, and attenuated familial adenomatous polyposis. *MUTYH* mutations are the cause of autosomal recessive *MUTYH*-associated polyposis syndrome. Although a number of clinical guidelines have been proposed to differentiate these conditions, it can still be very difficult to get an accurate and early diagnosis. The most common diagnostic problem lies in differentiating attenuated familial adenomatous polyposis and Lynch syndrome. The most common diagnostic approach to Lynch syndrome starts with tumor-based screening tests. This includes testing for microsatellite instability (MSI) and using immunohistochemistry to check for protein expression. However, these tests have false negatives. No tumor-based testing is available for polyposis syndromes.

An NGS panel, ColoSeq, is being offered clinically for such clinical scenarios where a clear diagnosis of hereditary colon cancer cannot be established (Pritchard et al. 2012). Technically, targeted capture and NGS on the Illumina HiSeq 2000 instrument was performed. The test assesses for single nucleotide and deletion/duplication analysis of mutations in *MLH1*, *MSH2*, *MSH6*, *PMS2*, *EPCAM*, *APC*, and *MUTYH*. In blinded specimens and colon cancer cell lines with defined mutations, ColoSeq correctly identified 28/28 (100 %) pathogenic mutations. This panel now includes additional genes such as *CDH1*, *PTEN*, *STK11*, *TP53*, *SMAD4*, and *BMPR1A*. The increase in gene number demonstrates the flexibility with respect to panel size and such panel expansion is necessary as genes become newly associated with diseases. Moreover, to increase the clinical sensitivity of this panel, deletion/duplication analysis of individual genes has been added. ColoSeq offers a powerful, cost-effective means of genetic testing for Lynch and polyposis syndromes that eliminates the need for stepwise testing and multiple follow-up clinical visits.

4.4   Mitochondrial Diseases

Mitochondrial diseases have the most varied presentation. This is because of the unique inheritance pattern of mitochondrial diseases. They can originate from mutations in either the nuclear or mitochondrial genome (Calvo et al. 2012). Their estimated prevalence is 1 in 5,000. Clinical presentation is usually as a primary skeletal and cardiomyopathy, neurologic disease, or multisystem disorder. Initial investigation may include blood and/or CSF lactate concentration, neuroimaging, cardiac evaluation, and muscle biopsy for histologic or histochemical evidence of mitochondrial disease. If a specific phenotype has been recognized, such as Leber hereditary optic neuropathy (LHON), Kearns–Sayre syndrome (KSS), chronic progressive external ophthalmoplegia (CPEO), mitochondrial encephalomyopathy with lactic acidosis and stroke-like episodes (MELAS), myoclonic epilepsy with ragged-red fibers (MERRF), neurogenic weakness with ataxia and retinitis pigmentosa (NARP), or Leigh syndrome (LS), the diagnosis can be confirmed by molecular genetic testing.

Approximately 70 nuclear genes have been implicated in mitochondrial diseases. However, many other genes are unknown. Mutations in mtDNA are suspected to cause adult onset disease. Mutations in nDNA usually cause pediatric disease. As the more common presentation of mitochondrial disease can be very nonspecific, it makes sense to test for mutations in both mtDNA and nDNA. However, traditional Sanger sequencing makes the cost very prohibitive. Hence NGS, which allows parallel sequencing, can dramatically reduce cost (Calvo et al. 2012). To explore its diagnostic use, a mitochondrial gene panel consisting of all the mitochondrial genome and additional 1,000 nuclear genes was assessed by examining 42 unrelated infants with clinical and biochemical evidence of mitochondrial oxidative phosphorylation disease (Vasta et al. 2009). In total, 23 of 42 (55 %) patients harbored mutations in recessive genes or pathogenic mtDNA variants. Firm diagnoses were enabled in ten patients (24 %) who had mutations in genes previously linked to disease. Thirteen patients (31 %) had mutations in nuclear genes not previously linked to disease. The results underscore the potential and challenges of deploying NGS in clinical settings.

4.5 Cardiovascular Diseases

The impact of NGS on inherited cardiomyopathies is tremendous (Meder et al. 2011). The major clinical forms of inherited cardiomyopathy are hypertrophic (HCM) and dilated (DCM; Meder et al. 2011). HCM usually presents as a sudden cardiac death and is a major cause of morbidity in young people and it can also cause heart failure. It presents with a left ventricular hypertrophy, usually asymmetric. Functionally, it causes diastolic dysfunction and histologically it can show up as myofibrillar disarray. In contrast, dilated cardiomyopathy is manifested as diastolic dysfunction caused by dilated ventricular cavity, leading to heart failure as its most common manifestation. HCM is caused by mutation in genes responsible for sarcomere formation. More than 450 mutations have been identified in 16 genes (Meder et al. 2011). DCM is caused by mutations in genes encoding proteins in sarcomere, Z-disk, nuclear lamina proteins, intermediate filaments, and the glycoprotein complexes.

Meder et al. established a microarray-based subgenomic enrichment followed by NGS to detect mutations in patients with HCM and DCM (Meder et al. 2011). Interestingly, NGS sequencing of patients with an unknown genetic cause of cardiomyopathy were found to have well-known disease mutations for HCM or DCM. This approach allowed, for the first time, a comprehensive genetic screening in patients with hereditary DCM or HCM in a fast and cost-efficient manner.

A different set of cardiomyopathies is caused by defects in primary electrical conduction defects. The most common are the Brugada syndrome and Long QT (LQT) syndrome. Mutations are seen in sodium and potassium channels. Brugada syndrome is caused by mutations in eight genes (*CN5A*, *GPD1L*, *CACNA1C*, *CACNB2*, *SCN1B*, *KCNE3*, *SCN3B*, and *HCN4*). LQT syndrome genes are labeled *LQT1-13*. NGS has tremendous potential in shortening the diagnostic odyssey in these patients. In fact, several panels for these genes are commercially available by a number of clinical laboratories nationwide. These NGS tests include a 12-gene LQT syndrome panel, a nine-gene Brugada syndrome panel, and a 29-gene arrhythmia panel that incorporates genes implicated in LQT syndrome, Brugada, catecholaminergic polymorphic ventricular tachycardia and several other arrhythmic disorders, as well as sudden cardiac arrest.

Aortic root dilatations are another set of disorders for which NGS has already established itself in a clinical setting. Aortic root dilatation can be caused by a number of disorders such as Marfan syndrome (MFS), Loeys–Dietz syndrome, Ehlers–Danlos syndrome type IV, and congenital contractual arachnodactyly. In addition, nonsyndromic causes of aortic root dilatation include mutations in genes related to the structure and function of the aortic wall, including *MYH11*, *ACTA2*, *SLC2A10*, and *NOTCH1*. Commercial clinical laboratories offer a combination of any number of these genes on their NGS panels. For example, the Marfan, aneurysm, and related disorders NGS panel is a comprehensive gene sequencing test for ten genes (*ACTA2*, *CBS*, *FBN1*, *FBN2*, *MYH11*, *COL3A1*, *SLC2A10*, *SMAD3*, *TGFBR1*, and *TGFBR2*) associated with MFS and MFS-related disorders.

Familial cholesterolemia is caused by mutations in *LDLR* gene, Apo-lipoprotein B, and *PCSK9*. Clinically, it is important to identify the proband's mutation so that at-risk relatives can be recognized. Subsequently, at-risk individuals can be started on cholesterol lowering medications, as dietary modification will have no effect. NGS offers a fast and effective way to diagnose predisposing mutations in these disorders (Wooderchak-Donahue et al. 2012).

4.6 Ophthalmic Disorders

Mutations in more than 150 genes cause inherited retinal disorders, leading to a diversity of overlapping phenotypes. These diseases may be stationary (i.e., congenital stationary night blindness) or progressive (i.e., retinitis pigmentosa). These disorders may present by themselves, nonsyndromic, or as part of a syndromic disorder. To examine each individual gene is time-consuming and cost-prohibitive. Audo et al. established a solution capture (Agilent SureSelect, SS) and Genome Analyzer IIx (Illumina) approach to examine a 1,177 Mb region of interest against 254 known and candidate retinal disease genes (Audo et al. 2012). Their patients had phenotypes that included retinitis pigmentosa, congenital stationary night blindness, Best disease, early-onset cone dystrophy, and Stargardt disease. Interestingly, three known and five novel mutations were identified in *NR2E3*, *PRPF3*, *EYS*, *PRPF8*, *CRB1*, *TRPM1*, and *CACNA1F*. This unbiased NGS approach allowed mutation detection in 75 % of control cases and in 57 % of test cases. Authors found this approach to be time-efficient as well as novel because it allowed the possibility of expanding the phenotypes of known gene mutations.

Daiger et al. discuss the development of a VisionCHIP for autosomal dominant retinitis pigmentosa, which contains 593 genes, to address the issues of genetic heterogeneity. The selected genes were from the RetNet database of retinal disease genes as well as EyeSAGE database (Daiger et al. 2010). In this approach, a microarray with oligonucleotides was chosen to capture sheared human DNA, and eluted DNA was sequenced by NGS technology. To optimize and validate the VisionCHIP, the focus was on the usage of controls with known adRP mutations, including deletions, and on 21 families from the adRP cohort without known mutations. This approach may identify new RP genes and will substantially reduce the cost per patient.

4.7 Hematological Disorders

Primary immunodeficiencies are fast becoming highlights for policy makers as SCID is being added to newborn screening in various states in the United States. Missing or deregulated pathways in the immunological response cascade character-ize these disorders (Ghosh et al. 2012). The clinical presentations tend to be very similar and, for this reason, diagnosis is challenging. Some traditional techniques revolve around cytological testing, but cases can be missed. Ghosh et al. designed a custom microarray to capture exons of 395 human genes, known or predicted to be associated with primary immunodeficiency and immune regulation, and sequenced on a GS FLX Titanium 454 platform (Ghosh et al. 2012). Sequencing yielded 152,000–397,000 high-quality reads per patient with coverage of 76–82 % at 5X. Importantly, this approach found the genetic mutations in two patients with sus-pected primary immunodeficiency.

Similar to primary immunodeficiency, platelet function disorders (PFDs) are genotypically diverse but present with excessive mucocutaneous bleeding. Functionally assays may point towards a bleeding diathesis; however, they cannot pinpoint towards an accurate genetic cause. Jones et al. describe a strategy for genetic diagnosis of PFDs with Agilent SS in-solution enrichment and Illumina sequencing of 216 candidate genes (Jones et al. 2012). A candidate list of genes includes *HPS1*, *HPS1*, *VPS33B*, *NAPA*, *LYST*, *HPS4*, *VPS18*, *VPS16*, *SCL3n*, and *HPS4* (Jones et al. 2012). In ten subjects, approximately 4,500 potential variants, in the 216 candidate genes, were filtered to a shortlist of ten potentially pathogenic variants. This proof-of-principle study illustrates that NGS enables rapid genetic diagnosis of a PFD in a single test.

4.8   Primary Ciliary Dyskinesia

These are autosomal recessive disorders characterized by abnormalities of motile cilia, which result in phenotypes ranging and including situs inversus, neonatal respiratory distress at full-term birth, recurrent otitis media, chronic sinusitis, chronic bronchitis that may result in bronchiectasis, and male infertility. It can be caused by mutations in nine different genes (*DNAH5*, *DNAH11*, *DNAI1*, *DNAI2*, *KTU*, *LRRC50*, *RSPH9*, *RSPH4A*, and *TXNDC3*). Immunohistochemistry can be used to detect loss of specific proteins as these disorders have defective dynein arms or other axonemal components, but this will not point towards a specific genetic etiology. Hence multiplexing on an NGS platform is highly desirable (Berg et al. 2011). A pilot study of four individuals with primary ciliary dyskinesia mutations was conducted using a custom array (NimbleGen), to capture 2,089 exons from 79 genes associated with primary ciliary dyskinesia or ciliary function, and sequencing was performed on the GS FLX Titanium (Roche 454) platform. Three out of three substitution mutations and one of three small insertion/deletion mutations were readily identified using this methodology. Importantly, this process failed to detect two known mutations: one single-nucleotide insertion and a whole-exon deletion.

Similar to primary ciliary dysplasia are the nephronophthisis-associated ciliopathies (NPHP-AC; Otto et al. 2011). These comprise a group of autosomal recessive cystic kidney diseases that includes nephronophthisis (NPHP), Senior–Loken syndrome (SLS), Joubert syndrome (JBTS), and Meckel–Gruber syndrome (MKS). Just like PCD, a number of genes have been implicated in NPHP-AC (*NPHP1*, *INVS*, *NPHP3*, *NPHP4*, *IQCB1*, *CEP290*, *GLIS2*, *RPGRIP1L*, *NEK8*, *TMEM67*, *INPP5E*, *TMEM216*, *AHI1*, *ARL13B*, *CC2D2A*, *TTC21B*, *MKS1*, and *XPNPEP3*). Otto et al. examined 120 patients with severe NPHP-AC phenotypes by PCR amplifying all 376 exons of 18 NPHP-AC genes and subjecting the amplicons to sequencing on Illumina Genome Analyzer. DNA from patients with known mutations were used and detection of 22 out of 24 different alleles (92 % sensitivity) was demonstrated. NGS led to the molecular diagnosis in 30/120 patients (25 %) and 54 pathogenic mutations (27 novel) were identified in seven different NPHP-AC genes.

4.9   Urea Cycle Disorders

Urea cycle disorders (UCDs) are caused by defects in the enzymes, which are involved in the transfer of nitrogen from ammonia to urea. This can lead to toxic hyperammonemia. There are a total of six genes involved in coding for six enzymes, which include carbamoylphosphate synthetase I (CPS1), ornithine transcarbamylase (OTC), argininosuccinic acid synthetase (ASS1), argininosuccinic acid lyase (ASL), arginase (ARG), and *N*-acetyl glutamate synthetase (NAGS). Biochemical analysis of intermediary metabolites (plasma amino acids and urine orotic acid) is used to diagnose inborn UCDs and genetic mutation testing is commonly used to confirm diagnosis. However, there are certain limitations to this approach. Deleterious mutations located deep within the introns of the OTC gene are typically not scanned by Sanger sequencing in clinical laboratories. In addition, larger genes are also involved making diagnosis time-consuming, and, sometimes, biochemically it is difficult to distinguish between NAGS and CPS1 deficiencies. Ambiguous results can also be seen in late-onset forms of OTC deficiency. NGS was shown to play an important role in screening for multiple genes and improves diagnostic efficiency (Amstutz et al. 2011). In a study of UCD, a custom array and a 454 sequencer were used to examine variants in three genes of four patients (Amstutz et al. 2011). Heterozygous and homozygous disease-associated mutations were correctly detected in all samples.

4.10 Summary

As NGS technologies develop, we will have the ability to generate large amounts of sequence data at lower cost and with less effort. This will eventually lead to improved diagnosis of heterogeneous disorders. In the past few years, the translation of NGS to the clinical realm has been steadily increasing. NGS technologies have been applied to the examination of a large number of genes in numerous genetically heterogeneous disorders, as well as genes from one common pathway. We expect the applications of NGS to continue to expand and to encompass other areas of medicine as focused panel tests, a whole exome test, and, in the near future, a whole genome test.

References

Amstutz U, Andrey-Zürcher G, Suciu D et al (2011) Sequence capture and next-generation resequencing of multiple tagged nucleic acid samples for mutation screening of urea cycle disorders. Clin Chem 57:102–111. doi:10.1373/clinchem.2010.150706

Audo I, Bujakowska KM, Léveillard T et al (2012) Development and application of a next-generation-sequencing (NGS) approach to detect known and novel gene defects underlying retinal diseases. Orphanet J Rare Dis 7:8. doi:10.1186/1750-1172-7-8

Berg JS, Evans JP, Leigh MW et al (2011) Next generation massively parallel sequencing of targeted exomes to identify genetic mutations in primary ciliary dyskinesia: implications for application to clinical testing. Genet Med 13:218–229. doi:10.1097/GIM.0b013e318203cff2

Calvo SE, Compton AG, Hershman SG et al (2012) Molecular diagnosis of infantile mitochondrial disease with targeted next-generation sequencing. Sci Transl Med 4:118ra10. doi:10.1126/scitranslmed.3003310

Chan M, Ji SM, Yeo ZX et al (2012) Development of a next-generation sequencing method for BRCA mutation screening: a comparison between a high-throughput and a benchtop platform. J Mol Diagn 14:602–612. doi:10.1016/j.jmoldx.2012.06.003

Chiu RWK, Chan KCA, Gao Y et al (2008) Noninvasive prenatal diagnosis of fetal chromosomal aneuploidy by massively parallel genomic sequencing of DNA in maternal plasma. Proc Natl Acad Sci U S A 105:20458–20463. doi:10.1073/pnas.0810641105

Daiger SP, Sullivan LS, Bowne SJ et al (2010) Targeted high-throughput DNA sequencing for gene discovery in retinitis pigmentosa. Adv Exp Med Biol 664:325–331. doi:10.1007/978-1-4419-1399-9_37

Ghosh S, Krux F, Binder V et al (2012) Array-based sequence capture and next-generation sequencing for the identification of primary immunodeficiencies. Scand J Immunol 75: 350–354. doi:10.1111/j.1365-3083.2011.02658.x

Hoischen A, Gilissen C, Arts P et al (2010) Massively parallel sequencing of ataxia genes after array-based enrichment. Hum Mutat 31:494–499. doi:10.1002/humu.21221

Hu H, Wrogemann K, Kalscheuer V et al (2009) Mutation screening in 86 known X-linked mental retardation genes by droplet-based multiplex PCR and massive parallel sequencing. HUGO J 3:41–49. doi:10.1007/s11568-010-9137-y

Jones MA, Bhide S, Chin E et al (2011) Targeted polymerase chain reaction-based enrichment and next-generation sequencing for diagnostic testing of congenital disorders of glycosylation. Genet Med 13:921–932. doi:10.1097/GIM.0b013e318226fbf2

Jones ML, Murden SL, Bem D et al (2012) Rapid genetic diagnosis of heritable platelet function disorders with next-generation sequencing: proof-of-principle with Hermansky-Pudlak syndrome. J Thromb Haemost 10:306–309. doi:10.1111/j.1538-7836.2011.04569.x

Lim BC, Lee S, Shin J-Y et al (2011) Genetic diagnosis of Duchenne and Becker muscular dystrophy using next-generation sequencing technology: comprehensive mutational search in a single platform. J Med Genet 48:731–736. doi:10.1136/jmedgenet-2011-100133

Meder B, Haas J, Keller A et al (2011) Targeted next-generation sequencing for the molecular genetic diagnostics of cardiomyopathies. Circ Cardiovasc Genet 4:110–122. doi:10.1161/CIRCGENETICS.110.958322

Otto EA, Ramaswami G, Janssen S et al (2011) Mutation analysis of 18 nephronophthisis associated ciliopathy disease genes using a DNA pooling and next-generation sequencing strategy. J Med Genet 48:105–116. doi:10.1136/jmg.2010.082552

Pritchard CC, Smith C, Salipante SJ et al (2012) ColoSeq provides comprehensive lynch and polyposis syndrome mutational analysis using massively parallel sequencing. J Mol Diagn 14:357–366. doi:10.1016/j.jmoldx.2012.03.002

Rehman AU, Morell RJ, Belyantseva IA et al (2010) Targeted capture and next-generation sequencing identifies C9orf75, encoding taperin, as the mutated gene in nonsyndromic deafness DFNB79. Am J Hum Genet 86:378–388. doi:10.1016/j.ajhg.2010.01.030

Valencia CA, Rhodenizer D, Bhide S et al (2012) Assessment of target enrichment platforms using massively parallel sequencing for the mutation detection for congenital muscular dystrophy. J Mol Diagn 14:233–246. doi:10.1016/j.jmoldx.2012.01.009

Vasta V, Ng SB, Turner EH et al (2009) Next generation sequence analysis for mitochondrial disorders. Genome Med 1:100. doi:10.1186/gm100

Wooderchak-Donahue WL, O'Fallon B, Furtado LV et al (2012) A direct comparison of next-generation sequencing enrichment methods using an aortopathy gene panel—clinical diagnostics perspective. BMC Med Genomics 5:50. doi:10.1186/1755-8794-5-50

Chapter 5
Next-Generation–Sequencing-Based Noninvasive Prenatal Diagnosis

5.1 Introduction

Prenatal diagnosis is important part of obstetric practice (Tounta et al. 2011). Traditionally, fetal DNA is obtained by invasive techniques, namely, amniocentesis and chorionic villus sampling. Such invasive procedure leads to a miscarriage rate of about 1 % and is reserved only for high risk pregnancies for specific genetic conditions which include fetal chromosomal aneuploidies and monogenic disorders with relatively high prevalence in the relevant populations. The ultimate goal for early prenatal diagnosis, while decreasing the miscarriage rate, is to employ noninvasive testing using maternal peripheral blood as a source of fetal genetic material (Tounta et al. 2011). Multiple studies indicate that both intact fetal cells and cell-free fetal nucleic acids (cffNA) cross the placenta and can be found in the maternal circulation. Intact fetal cells present an attractive target for noninvasive prenatal diagnosis (NIPD) of fetal chromosomal abnormalities (Lo et al. 1996). Isolation and analysis of fetal cells from maternal circulation have been extensively investigated and several methods for fetal cell enrichment have been developed (Bianchi 1999; Jackson 2003; Sekizawa et al. 2007). However, due to the lack of cells in the maternal circulation and low efficiency of enrichment methods results have not been promising. In addition, it has been challenging to perform Fluorescent In Situ Hybridization (FISH) because of the presence of apoptotic nuclei of fetal cells (Bianchi et al. 1997).

In 1997, Lo et al. reported the presence of cell-free fetal DNA (cffDNA) in maternal plasma and serum in amounts significantly increased, as compared to fetal DNA extracted from the cellular fraction of maternal blood (Lo et al. 1997). This discovery rapidly paved the way for the detection of paternally inherited alleles in maternal blood, including, most notably, Rh D blood group, fetal sex, and single-gene disorders. For more than a decade now, NIPD has been used routinely for pregnancies in which paternally inherited alleles require detection because their inheritance would indicate a clinical condition, such as hemolytic disease of the fetus and newborn, congenital adrenal hyperplasia, and hemophilia (Avent et al.

C.A. Valencia et al., *Next Generation Sequencing Technologies in Medical Genetics*, SpringerBriefs in Genetics, DOI 10.1007/978-1-4614-9032-6_5, © C. Alexander Valencia 2013

2009; Avent and Chitty 2006; Bianchi et al. 2005; Hahn et al. 2011; van der Schoot et al. 2003). NIPD has been more challenging for conditions in which analysis of maternal alleles is required owing to the ubiquitous presence of free maternal DNA in plasma. This situation still represents the most important technical obstacle to achieving routine NIPD for the common chromosomal abnormalities, such as aneuploidy.

In 2008, however, there appeared a brace of reports that applied the emerging next-generation–sequencing (NGS) technologies to the analysis of trisomies with DNA extracted from maternal plasma (Chiu et al. 2008; Fan et al. 2008). Several groups confirmed this breakthrough, and last years investigation of a very large cohort proved the efficacy of NGS as applied to chromosome counting in maternal plasma samples (Chiu et al. 2011). Several consortia [e.g., the European Commission consortium EuroGentest (http://www.eurogentest.org) and the UK RAPID consortium (http://www.rapid.nhs.uk)] are driving the implementation of this technology into clinical practice. Thus, in this chapter we explore the exquisite resolution of NGS and its ability to sequence a population of DNA molecules to define chromosome copy number following the introduction of the common aneuploidy T21.

5.2   Trisomy 21, a Common Aneuploidy

Trisomy 21 (T21) is the most common chromosomal abnormality in live-born children. By employing invasive testing, the diagnosis can be determined early in pregnancy with a high risk of miscarriage (Lo et al. 2007). These tests are routinely for women at increased risk for fetal trisomy based on maternal age, serum markers for trisomy, and ultrasound measurement of the fetal nuchal translucency (Driscoll et al. 2009). From screening program data, one in every 20 women is offered invasive testing (Wapner et al. 2003). Recently, NIPD, through the use of cffDNA, has been employed to the diagnosis of T21 (Lo et al. 2007). However, due to the variability (1–10 %) of percentage of cffDNA in maternal plasma, it remains challenging to detect fetal sequences in a large pool of maternal DNA (Hahn et al. 2011). Therefore, a number of methods have been developed and used in the field of noninvasive T21, including the NGS, and are described in the following section.

5.3   Methods for the Detection of cffDNA

The scarcity of cffDNA in maternal blood and its coexistence with maternal DNA represent the two major limitations for the use of cffDNA for diagnosis. Both maternal plasma and serum contain cffDNA; however, plasma is the material of choice for prenatal diagnosis since it contains less maternal background DNA. Various methods have been used to overcome the presence of maternal background cell-free DNA (cfDNA), including methods based on the size difference of maternal fragments (Chan et al. 2004). Efforts to increase the relative proportion of fetal DNA compared to the larger maternal fraction have also included the use of form-aldehyde, as a fixative, to prevent lysis of maternal cells during the isolation of the maternal plasma (Dhallan et al. 2004). The formaldehyde enrichment technique, however, has not been reproducible by other laboratories.

Different methodologies applied for the detection of cffDNA include conventional PCR, restriction analysis, quantitative fluorescence real-time PCR (QF-PCR), and automated sequencing (Bustamante-Aragones et al. 2008; Chiu et al. 2002a, b; Ding et al. 2004; Li et al. 2007; Saito et al. 2000). Since QF-PCR is more sensitive compared to conventional PCR, enabling the detection of very low copy numbers of DNA, it represents the optimal method for reliable NIPD. The main advantage of QF-PCR is that it is quantitative and collects data in the exponential growth phase of the reaction, which is the most specific and precise one. The technique is less time-consuming and offers an extra level of protection against contamination. A wide range of Ct values in each QF-PCR and poor repeatability of some replicates are reported, partly due to the variability of target copy number in maternal plasma. It is, therefore, recommended to perform several replicates from each maternal sample in order to increase the probability of fetal DNA detection and to avoid false negative results (Minon et al. 2008). Recently, new sophisticated molecular techniques, such as NGS, have emerged and have been applied to the field of NIPD (Fan et al. 2008). They have higher sensitivity, but the expensive and complicated handling processes are required by these techniques. NGS can analyze the nucleotide sequences of millions of DNA molecules in each run. The capacity of NGS to differentiate small quantitative alterations in genomic distributions of chromosomes has allowed detection of higher number of chromosome 21 sequences in trisomy 21 pregnancies as compared to euploid pregnancies.

5.4   Principle of Aneuploidy Detection with Next-Generation–Sequencing

The principle of the use of NGS for noninvasive fetal chromosomal aneuploidy detection in maternal plasma is shown in Fig. 5.1 (Chiu et al. 2008). Maternal plasma DNA (maternal and fetal) is naturally fragmented and further fragmentation is unnecessary for the next steps (Chan et al. 2004). The plasma DNA fragments are sequenced by an Illumina sequencer and processed by the Efficient Large-Scale Alignment of Nucleotide Databases (ELAND) software to determine the chromosomal origin, but the details about their gene-specific location are not required. Quantification of the number of sequence reads originating from any particular chromosome is performed for each human chromosome. Chiu et al. counted only sequences that could be mapped to just one location, unique sequences denoted as U0–1–0–0 on the basis of values in a number of fields in the data output files of the ELAND sequence alignment software, in the repeat-masked reference human genome with no mismatch. The percentage contribution of unique sequences

Fig. 5.1 Schematic
illustration for the
noninvasive prenatal
detection of fetal
chromosomal aneuploidy
using next-generation–
sequencing (adapted from
Chiu et al. 2008)

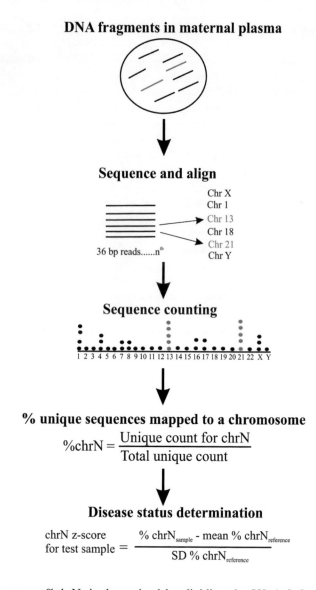

DNA fragments in maternal plasma

Sequence and align

Chr X
Chr 1
Chr 13
Chr 18
Chr 21
Chr Y

36 bp reads......nth

Sequence counting

1 2 3 4 5 6 7 8 9 10 11 12 13 14 15 16 17 18 19 20 21 22 X Y

% unique sequences mapped to a chromosome

$$\%chrN = \frac{\text{Unique count for chrN}}{\text{Total unique count}}$$

Disease status determination

$$\text{chrN z-score for test sample} = \frac{\%\ chrN_{sample} - mean\ \%\ chrN_{reference}}{SD\ \%\ chrN_{reference}}$$

mapped to each chromosome, %chrN, is determined by dividing the U0–1–0–0 count of a specific chromosome by the total number of U0–1–0–0 sequence reads generated in the sequencing run for the tested sample. Then, the z-score, defined as the number of standard deviations from the mean of a reference data set, of %chr21 of the tested sample is calculated to determine whether or not it was a T21 pregnancy. Hence, for a T21 fetus, a high z-score for %chr21 is expected when compared with the mean and standard deviation of %chr21 values obtained from maternal plasma of euploid pregnancies.

Despite the potential applications of the method, it is important to be aware of the assumptions that are made for effective noninvasive prenatal fetal chromosomal aneuploidy detection and specifically the %chrN values should be reflective of the genomic representation of the maternal and fetal DNA fragments in maternal plasma. NGS must permit capture and sequencing of the small fetal DNA fraction alongside the maternal DNA. Moreover, the captured and sequenced pool of plasma DNA must represent the total DNA pool with similar interchromosomal distribution to that in the original maternal plasma. In addition, a minimal bias in ability to sequence DNA fragments originating from each chromosome is assumed. Furthermore, if both the maternal and the fetal genomes are evenly represented in maternal plasma, the proportional contribution of plasma DNA sequences per chromosome should in turn bear correlation with the relative size of each chromosome in the human genome.

5.5   Noninvasive Diagnosis of Fetal Aneuploidy by Shotgun Sequencing DNA

Fan et al. applied NGS on cfDNA from plasma of pregnant women with a gestational age of 10–35 weeks (Fan et al. 2008). They directly sequenced cfDNA with a high-throughput shotgun sequencing technology (Illumina's platform) and obtained five million sequence tags per patient from plasma of 18 pregnant women. An average of 154,000, 135,000, and 65,700 sequence tags mapped to chromosomes 13, 18, and 21 were obtained, respectively. This enabled the measurement of over- and underrepresentation of chromosomes from an aneuploid fetus. The distribution of chromosome 21 sequence tag density for all nine T21 pregnancies was clearly separated from that of pregnancies bearing disomy 21 fetuses. The coverage of chromosome 21 for T21 cases was 4–18 % higher (average 11 %) than that of the disomy 21 cases. Moreover, plasma DNA of pregnant women carrying T18 fetuses (two cases) and a T13 fetus (one case) were also directly sequenced. Overrepresentation was observed for chromosomes 18 and 13 in T18 and T13 cases, respectively. Although there were not enough positive samples to measure a representative distribution, it was encouraging that all of these three positives were outliers from the distribution of disomy values. The T18 were large outliers and were clearly statistically significant, whereas the statistical significance of the single T13 case was marginal. An advantage of using direct sequencing to measure aneuploidy noninvasively is that it is able to make full use of the sample, whereas PCR-based methods analyze only a few targeted sequences. Fan et al. showed successful development of a truly universal, polymorphism-independent noninvasive test for fetal aneuploidy. The sequencing approach is polymorphism-independent and therefore universally applicable for the noninvasive detection of fetal aneuploidy. Using this method, authors successfully identified all nine cases of trisomy 21 (Down syndrome), two cases of trisomy 18 (Edward syndrome), and one case of trisomy 13 (Patau syndrome) in a cohort of 18 normal and aneuploid pregnancies; trisomy was detected at gestational ages as early as the 14th week. Direct sequencing also allowed the study of the characteristics of cell-free plasma DNA, and evidence was found that this DNA is enriched for sequences from nucleosomes.

5.6 Noninvasive Prenatal Diagnosis of Fetal Chromosomal Aneuploidy by Next-Generation–Sequencing

Chiu et al. applied the same technique as Fan et al., but followed a different strategy for data analysis (Chiu et al. 2008). They used this strategy in order to detect trisomy 21. They tested an algorithm to calculate the percentage of unique sequences for the chromosome of interest in the test sample and compared it with the reference population of that same chromosome. The differences in amounts of chr21 DNA sequences in maternal plasma contributed by T21 fetuses compared with euploid fetuses were unambiguously demonstrated due to the ability of NGS to sequence a large number of molecules. For example, about ten million 36-bp reads were generated for each plasma sample, which was equivalent to just one-tenth of the human genome. Furthermore, in this study, only the U0–1–0–0 sequences, representing just 20 % of all of the reads sequenced from each plasma DNA sample, were used to generate a quantitative profile of chromosomal distribution. In contrast to previous methods that relied on coverage quantification, this method simply sequences a random representative fraction of the human genome. The relative chromosome size is then deduced by counting the relative number of sequences aligned to the chromosome. Despite the randomness of the sequencing, the quantitative estimation of %chr21 sequences was so precise and robust that the z-scores for chr21 of the T21 pregnancies were markedly different from the mean of a reference euploid sample set. Similarly, absolute differences in amounts of chrX and chrY DNA sequences in maternal plasma contributed by male fetuses compared with female fetuses were convincingly observed. Measurements of the genomic representations for chromosomes 13 and 18 were less precise (Chiu et al. 2010). The important advantage of the NGS technique is that it is gender- and polymorphism-independent, applicable in all pregnancies and likely to allow analysis of all frequent forms of aneuploidies in the same test. Currently, the technique is technically demanding, the cost per tested sample is high, and the throughput per instrument is low (16 samples per week). This prevents its use as a regular test for all pregnant women. Recently, three large-scale clinical studies were published showing results that NGS of maternal DNA of pregnant women is a powerful molecular diagnostic tool for diagnosis of fetal aneuploidies (Chiu et al. 2011; Ehrich et al. 2011; Palomaki et al. 2011). Furthermore, it was shown that NGS in combination with targeted enrichment of chromosome X is also a suitable approach for noninvasive detection of fetal-specific alleles (Liao et al. 2011).

5.7 Noninvasive Prenatal Diagnosis of Fetal Chromosomal Aneuploidy Using Different Next-Generation– Sequencing Strategies and Algorithms

Stumm et al. tested whether other sequencing and enrichment platforms could be used for NIPD of fetal chromosomal aneuploidy (Stumm et al. 2012). Specifically, they showed the ability to adopt various NGS technologies and to provide new algorithms for the quantification of fetal aneuploidies. Clearly, NGS was successfully applied for the detection of fetal trisomy 21. The study focused on sequencing 42 samples using the GAIIx and sequencing of 38 samples using the HiSeq 2000. On the basis of the algorithm hg18_rm_0mm for z-score calculation described by Chiu et al. all trisomy 21 samples were identified. Furthermore, the power of quantification detection of trisomy 21 was improved by establishing new algorithms to calculate the z-score. The algorithm hg18_par_X_Y_0mm_autosomes based on using only UMR-0mm of autosomes was the most suitable calculation method for this assay. In addition, for the first time a combination of the 38 Mb SureSelect Human All Exome target enrichment system followed by sequencing allowed the identification of fetal trisomy 13 and fetal trisomy 21. However, further studies are necessary to prove that it might be an alternative approach to detect all chromosomal aneuploidies.

5.8 Single Molecule Sequencing for the Detection of Trisomy 21

van den Oever et al. described the application of single molecule NGS (with the Helicos BioSciences platform) to the detection of trisomy 21 (van den Oever et al. 2012). NGS has developed substantially over the past 5 years, but most platforms require the preliminary amplification of genomic DNA sequences which introduces sequence-specific artifacts. Single molecule NGS bypasses this requirement, and the authors have compared the efficacy of this approach with that of amplification-based NGS (Illumina's Genome Analyzer II) by using identical maternal plasma samples obtained from mothers with (control) euploid and trisomy 21 fetuses. The Helicos platform uses visual imaging across the flow cell for direct DNA measurement by recording the incorporation of fluorescently labeled nucleotides (Milos 2009). This approach largely overcomes the limitations associated with PCR amplification and bias. The sequencing time on the Helicos platform is longer (4 vs. 2 days, respectively), sample preparation is simple, relatively inexpensive, and requires a low DNA input compared to Illumina.

A successful fetal T21 detection using free DNA from maternal plasma by single molecule sequencing on the Helicos platform was demonstrated (van den Oever et al. 2012). The greater sensitivity achieved with this platform is clearly advantageous because it permits early diagnosis, which the authors of this study reported being successful as early as 9 weeks, 3 days gestation. In addition, the Helicos platform is not biased in GC-rich areas, thereby leading to increased accuracy of analysis compared to the Illumina platform. This study shows for the first time that single molecule sequencing can be a reliable and easy-to-use alternative for noninvasive T21 detection in diagnostics. By using single molecule sequencing, previously described experimental noise associated with PCR amplification, such as GC bias, can be overcome. The work clearly shows that further refinement of NGS will pave the way for routine use of NIPD for aneuploidy.

5.9   Factors Affecting Next-Generations–Sequencing for Aneuploidy Determination

The average fetal fraction in maternal plasma is typically 10–15 %, but the range is from less than 3 % to greater than 30 % (Canick et al. 2013). Screening performance using NGS is less reliable in samples whose values are less than 3 %. There are three factors that affect the clinical fetal fraction for the application of aneuploidy diagnosis (Canick et al. 2013). As expected, as the fetal fraction increases the results for Down syndrome clearly improve. Second, the strongest factor associated with fetal fraction is maternal weight; the false negative rate and rate of low fetal fractions are highest for women with high maternal weights. Third, in a mosaic, the degree of mosaicism will impact the performance of the test, because it will reduce the effective fetal fraction. By understanding these aspects of the role of fetal fraction in maternal plasma DNA testing for aneuploidy, we can better appreciate the power and the limitations of this impressive new methodology (Canick et al. 2013).

5.10   Limitations of Noninvasive Prenatal Screening

The advent of prenatal genetic diagnosis is a major breakthrough, initially by amniocentesis in the second trimester of pregnancy and subsequently by chorionic villus sampling during the first trimester (Noninvasive Prenatal Screening Work Group of the American College of Medical Genetics and Genomics et al. 2013). Fetal loss due to invasive procedures has driven the search for noninvasive approaches for genetic screening and diagnosis. Typically, noninvasive screening for aneuploidy was performed by measuring maternal serum analytes and/or ultrasonography with positive screen rates of ~5 % and detection rates of 50–95 %, depending on the screening strategy utilized. Recently, genomic technologies have resulted in the development of a noninvasive prenatal screening (NIPS) test using cffDNA sequences isolated from a maternal blood sample. Thus far, studies have shown high sensitivity and specificity with low false-positive rates; however, there are limitations to NIPS. For example, the specificity and sensitivity are not uniform for all chromosomes which may result in false positives (Chen et al. 2011). Another issue is that the sequences are derived from the placenta and may not dictate the true fetal karyotype. Therefore, invasive testing for confirmation of a positive screening test should remain an option for patients seeking a definitive diagnosis (Noninvasive Prenatal Screening Work Group of the American College of Medical Genetics and Genomics et al. 2013).

The American College of Medical Genetics and Genomics published a statement on NIPS for fetal aneuploidy and points out the following limitations (Noninvasive Prenatal Screening Work Group of the American College of Medical Genetics and Genomics et al. 2013):

1. Risk assessment is limited to specific fetal aneuploidies (trisomy 13, 18, and 21) at this time.

2. Chromosomal abnormalities such as unbalanced translocations, deletions, and duplications will not be detected by NIPS.
3. NIPS is not able to distinguish specific forms of aneuploidy. For example, NIPS cannot determine if Down syndrome is due to the presence of an extra chromosome (trisomy 21), a Robertsonian translocation involving chromosome 21, or high-level mosaicism.
4. NIPS does not screen for single-gene mutations.
5. Uninformative test results due to insufficient isolation of cffDNA could lead to a delay in diagnosis or eliminate the availability of information for risk assessment.
6. Currently, it takes longer for NIPS test results to be returned than for test results on maternal serum analytes.
7. NIPS does not screen for open neural tube defects.
8. NIPS does not replace the utility of a first-trimester ultrasound examination, which has been proven to be useful for accurate gestational dating, assessment of the nuchal translucency region to identify a fetus at increased risk for a chromosome abnormality, identification of twins and higher-order pregnancies, placental abnormalities, and congenital anomalies.
9. Limited data are currently available on the use of NIPS in twins and higher-order pregnancies.
10. NIPS has no role in predicting late-pregnancy complications.

5.11   Summary

NGS technologies have been applied to the analysis of trisomies, namely, T21, T18, and T13, with DNA extracted from maternal plasma (Chiu et al. 2008; Fan et al. 2008). Importantly, large cohort studies proved the efficacy of NGS as applied to chromosome counting in maternal plasma samples (Chiu et al. 2011). Improvements on the original method have been attempted by implementation of new analysis algorithms and exome enrichment technologies. Moreover, single molecule sequencing for the detection of trisomy 21 has been successfully demonstrated. Even though these are promising new methods, there are factors that affect aneuploidy determination by NGS including fetal fraction level, maternal weight, and mosaicism. In addition, there are a number of limitations of NIPS that the ACMG has described. Therefore, continued research and agreement among several consortia will determine the fate of this technology in clinical practice.

References

Avent ND, Chitty LS (2006) Non-invasive diagnosis of fetal sex; utilisation of free fetal DNA in maternal plasma and ultrasound. Prenat Diagn 26:598–603. doi:10.1002/pd.1493

Avent ND, Madgett TE, Maddocks DG, Soothill PW (2009) Cell-free fetal DNA in the maternal serum and plasma: current and evolving applications. Curr Opin Obstet Gynecol 21:175–179. doi:10.1097/GCO.0b013e3283294798

Bianchi DW (1999) Fetal cells in the maternal circulation: feasibility for prenatal diagnosis. Br J Haematol 105:574–583

Bianchi DW, Williams JM, Sullivan LM et al (1997) PCR quantitation of fetal cells in maternal blood in normal and aneuploid pregnancies. Am J Hum Genet 61:822–829. doi:10.1086/514885

Bianchi DW, Avent ND, Costa J-M, van der Schoot CE (2005) Noninvasive prenatal diagnosis of fetal Rhesus D: ready for Prime(r) Time. Obstet Gynecol 106:841–844. doi:10.1097/01. AOG.0000179477.59385.93

Bustamante-Aragones A, Gallego-Merlo J, Trujillo-Tiebas MJ et al (2008) New strategy for the prenatal detection/exclusion of paternal cystic fibrosis mutations in maternal plasma. J Cyst Fibros 7:505–510. doi:10.1016/j.jcf.2008.05.006

Canick JA, Palomaki GE, Kloza EM et al (2013) The impact of maternal plasma DNA fetal fraction on next-generation sequencing tests for common fetal aneuploidies. Prenat Diagn 33(7):667–674. doi:10.1002/pd.4126

Chan KCA, Zhang J, Hui ABY et al (2004) Size distributions of maternal and fetal DNA in maternal plasma. Clin Chem 50:88–92. doi:10.1373/clinchem.2003.024893

Chen EZ, Chiu RWK, Sun H et al (2011) Noninvasive prenatal diagnosis of fetal trisomy 18 and trisomy 13 by maternal plasma DNA sequencing. PLoS One 6:e21791. doi:10.1371/journal. pone.0021791

Chiu RWK, Lau TK, Cheung PT et al (2002a) Noninvasive prenatal exclusion of congenital adrenal hyperplasia by maternal plasma analysis: a feasibility study. Clin Chem 48:778–780

Chiu RWK, Lau TK, Leung TN et al (2002b) Prenatal exclusion of beta thalassaemia major by examination of maternal plasma. Lancet 360:998–1000

Chiu RWK, Chan KCA, Gao Y et al (2008) Noninvasive prenatal diagnosis of fetal chromosomal aneuploidy by massively parallel genomic sequencing of DNA in maternal plasma. Proc Natl Acad Sci U S A 105:20458–20463. doi:10.1073/pnas.0810641105

Chiu RWK, Sun H, Akolekar R et al (2010) Maternal plasma DNA analysis with massively parallel sequencing by ligation for noninvasive prenatal diagnosis of trisomy 21. Clin Chem 56:459–463. doi:10.1373/clinchem.2009.136507

Chiu RWK, Akolekar R, Zheng YWL et al (2011) Non-invasive prenatal assessment of trisomy 21 by multiplexed maternal plasma DNA sequencing: large scale validity study. BMJ 342:c7401

Dhallan R, Au W-C, Mattagajasingh S et al (2004) Methods to increase the percentage of free fetal DNA recovered from the maternal circulation. JAMA 291:1114–1119. doi:10.1001/jama. 291.9.1114

Ding C, Chiu RWK, Lau TK et al (2004) MS analysis of single-nucleotide differences in circulating nucleic acids: application to noninvasive prenatal diagnosis. Proc Natl Acad Sci U S A 101:10762–10767. doi:10.1073/pnas.0403962101

Driscoll DA, Gross SJ, Professional Practice Guidelines Committee (2009) Screening for fetal aneuploidy and neural tube defects. Genet Med 11:818–821. doi:10.1097/GIM.0b013e3181bb267b

Ehrich M, Deciu C, Zwiefelhofer T et al (2011) Noninvasive detection of fetal trisomy 21 by sequencing of DNA in maternal blood: a study in a clinical setting. Am J Obstet Gynecol 204:205.e1–11. doi:10.1016/j.ajog.2010.12.060

Fan HC, Blumenfeld YJ, Chitkara U et al (2008) Noninvasive diagnosis of fetal aneuploidy by shotgun sequencing DNA from maternal blood. Proc Natl Acad Sci U S A 105:16266–16271. doi:10.1073/pnas.0808319105

Hahn S, Lapaire O, Tercanli S et al (2011) Determination of fetal chromosome aberrations from fetal DNA in maternal blood: has the challenge finally been met? Expert Rev Mol Med 13:e16. doi:10.1017/S1462399411001852

Jackson L (2003) Fetal cells and DNA in maternal blood. Prenat Diagn 23:837–846. doi:10.1002/ pd.705

Li Y, Page-Christiaens GCML, Gille JJP et al (2007) Non-invasive prenatal detection of achondroplasia in size-fractionated cell-free DNA by MALDI-TOF MS assay. Prenat Diagn 27:11–17. doi:10.1002/pd.1608

Liao GJW, Lun FMF, Zheng YWL et al (2011) Targeted massively parallel sequencing of maternal plasma DNA permits efficient and unbiased detection of fetal alleles. Clin Chem 57:92–101. doi:10.1373/clinchem.2010.154336

Lo YM, Lo ES, Watson N et al (1996) Two-way cell traffic between mother and fetus: biologic and clinical implications. Blood 88:4390–4395

Lo YM, Corbetta N, Chamberlain PF et al (1997) Presence of fetal DNA in maternal plasma and serum. Lancet 350:485–487. doi:10.1016/S0140-6736(97)02174-0

Lo YMD, Tsui NBY, Chiu RWK et al (2007) Plasma placental RNA allelic ratio permits noninvasive prenatal chromosomal aneuploidy detection. Nat Med 13:218–223. doi:10.1038/nm1530

Milos PM (2009) Emergence of single-molecule sequencing and potential for molecular diagnostic applications. Expert Rev Mol Diagn 9:659–666. doi:10.1586/erm.09.50

Minon J-M, Gerard C, Senterre J-M et al (2008) Routine fetal RHD genotyping with maternal plasma: a four-year experience in Belgium. Transfusion 48:373–381. doi:10.1111/j.1537-2995.2007.01533.x

Noninvasive Prenatal Screening Work Group of the American College of Medical Genetics and Genomics, Gregg AR, Gross SJ et al (2013) ACMG statement on noninvasive prenatal screening for fetal aneuploidy. Genet Med 15:395–398. doi:10.1038/gim.2013.29

Palomaki GE, Kloza EM, Lambert-Messerlian GM et al (2011) DNA sequencing of maternal plasma to detect Down syndrome: an international clinical validation study. Genet Med 13:913–920. doi:10.1097/GIM.0b013e3182368a0e

Saito H, Sekizawa A, Morimoto T et al (2000) Prenatal DNA diagnosis of a single-gene disorder from maternal plasma. Lancet 356:1170. doi:10.1016/S0140-6736(00)02767-7

Sekizawa A, Purwosunu Y, Farina A et al (2007) Development of noninvasive fetal DNA diagnosis from nucleated erythrocytes circulating in maternal blood. Prenat Diagn 27:846–848. doi:10.1002/pd.1792

Stumm M, Entezami M, Trunk N et al (2012) Noninvasive prenatal detection of chromosomal aneuploidies using different next-generation sequencing strategies and algorithms. Prenat Diagn 32:569–577. doi:10.1002/pd.3862

Tounta G, Kolialexi A, Papantoniou N et al (2011) Non-invasive prenatal diagnosis using cell-free fetal nucleic acids in maternal plasma: progress overview beyond predictive and personalized diagnosis. EPMA J 2:163–171. doi:10.1007/s13167-011-0085-y

Van den Oever JME, Balkassmi S, Verweij EJ et al (2012) Single molecule sequencing of free DNA from maternal plasma for noninvasive trisomy 21 detection. Clin Chem 58:699–706. doi:10.1373/clinchem.2011.174698

Van der Schoot CE, Tax GHM, Rijnders RJP et al (2003) Prenatal typing of Rh and Kell blood group system antigens: the edge of a watershed. Transfus Med Rev 17:31–44. doi:10.1053/tmrv.2003.50001

Wapner R, Thom E, Simpson JL et al (2003) First-trimester screening for trisomies 21 and 18. N Engl J Med 349:1405–1413. doi:10.1056/NEJMoa025273

Chapter 6
Diagnosis of Inherited Neuromuscular Disorders by Next-Generation–Sequencing

6.1 Introduction

Inherited neuromuscular disorders (NMD) form a group of genetic diseases that result in long-term disability. The total incidence of NMD is greater than 1 in 3,000 and comprises a group of more than 200 monogenic disorders (Emery 1991). For about half of the cases, the molecular cause has not been identified. An extensive clinical evaluation with complementary gene-by-gene testing is often required to reach an exact diagnosis. Due to the presence of genetic heterogeneity and lack of segregation in sporatic cases, reaching a diagnosis is challenging, lengthy, and expensive. The genetic heterogeneity can be demonstrated by the number of genes involved in specific subgroups of NMD, namely, hereditary sensorimotor neuropathies (HSMN; 50 genes) and congenital muscular dystrophies (12 genes; North 2008; Valencia et al. 2013). In other instances, some NMD genes are very large and are not sequenced completely because it is costly and labor-intensive to sequence by the Sanger method. For the patient, this gene-by-gene approach increases the number of tests that are required, thus, delaying the diagnosis and exposing the patient to unnecessary investigations and treatments, precluding the full benefit of a targeted approach to treatment, and increasing recurrence risk in the families (Vasli et al. 2012).

Next-generation–sequencing (NGS) has been shown to interrogate multiple genes in parallel. This approach has been mainly used to identify novel disease genes in a research setting. Recently, several clinical laboratories, including Emory Genetics Laboratory (EGL) and Boston Children's DNA Diagnostic laboratories, have translated NGS and offer clinical muscular dystrophy panels. In the following sections, we summarize data that demonstrate the application of NGS to address genetic heterogeneity and large target sequencing intervals in NMD examples.

C.A. Valencia et al., *Next Generation Sequencing Technologies in Medical Genetics,*
SpringerBriefs in Genetics, DOI 10.1007/978-1-4614-9032-6_6,
© C. Alexander Valencia 2013

6.2 A Broad Neuromuscular Diseases Panel

A study reported the development of an efficient screening strategy for heterogeneous neuromuscular disease genes using two groups of patients; with or without known mutations (Vasli et al. 2012; Table 6.1). Solution-based targeted enrichment, Agilent SureSelect (SS) custom kit, of 267 known NMD genes (1.6 Mb target region) followed by NGS on an Illumina Genome Analyzer IIx was performed. After alignment with the human reference genome, the mean coverage of the targeted exons was 138X and the percentage of nucleotides with at least 10X coverage was 94 %. Most of the exons were captured (>97 %), but 168 exons had low coverage sequences due to high GC content. Mapping, variant calling, filtering, and ranking were used to prioritize variants. On average, 1,162 variants and 152 indels were identified, of which 341 were not reported as SNPs. In the NMD panel, on average 125 variants affecting splice sites or predicted to change the amino acid sequence were described. Further prioritization was based on VaRank, clinical phenotype, and segregation.

The challenge of NGS data analysis is the identification of the pathogenic changes among the large list of variants (Vasli et al. 2012). Significantly, the custom VaRank scoring program blindly ranked the known mutations and implicated genes first in the list based on disease class and inheritance mode. Importantly, clinical, histological, and molecular data were necessary for matching the genetic data with

Table 6.1 Capture and sequencing technologies that have been applied in the mutation detection of muscular dystrophies

Muscular dystrophy type(s)	No. of genes	No. of exons	Target interval (kbp)	Enrichment platform	NGS platform	Reference
Inherited neuromuscular disorders	267	4,604	1,600	Solution-based capture[a]	Illumina's Genome Analyzer IIx	Vasli et al. (2012)
Duchenne muscular dystrophy	1	79	30	Solid phase capture[b]	HiSeq 2000	Xie et al. (2012)
Congenital muscular dystrophies	12	321	65	RainDance[c], Solution-based capture[a]	SOLiD 3	Valencia et al. (2012)
Congenital muscular dystrophies	12	321	65	RainDance[c]	SOLiD 3	Valencia et al. (2013)
Duchenne muscular dystrophy, congenital muscular dystrophies, limb girdle muscular dystrophies	26	747	1,069	Solution-based capture[a]	Illumina's Genome Analyzer IIx	Lim et al. (2011)

[a]Solution-based capture, Agilent's hybridization-based SureSelect
[b]Solid phase capture, NimbleGen's hybridization-based microarray capture
[c]RainDance, highly multiplex PCR amplification

the phenotype. Moreover, this validation demonstrated that this approach can detect different mutation types in a wide range of heterogeneous diseases.

All the known and novel mutations were identified in previously characterized patients and in patients lacking molecular diagnosis (Vasli et al. 2012). Specifically, all mutation types, in the eight positive controls, were identified. The large deletion encompassing exons 18–44 of the *DMD* gene was detected in a patient with Duchenne muscular dystrophy by comparing the number of reads in these regions with other sequenced DNA samples. The mean coverage for exons 18–44 is 0X for this patient and 177X for other patients. Two mutations in *SETX* were found in two patients with ataxia. Similarly, samples from patients with heterogeneous NMD without molecular characterization were sequenced. Potential disease-causing mutations, supported by Sanger confirmation and segregation, were identified in several patients, namely, *RYR1*, *TTN*, and *COL6A3* (Vasli et al. 2012). These genes were also consistent with the clinical information. For example, compound heterozygous mutations were in the ryanodine receptor (*RYR1*) of a patient with muscular dystrophy and arthrogryposis. Additionally, the mutations were present in his affected twin brother and each parent was a carrier of each mutation.

NGS is suitable for analysis of diseases with high degree genetic heterogeneity with many potential candidate causative genes and allelic diseases caused by mutations of the same gene (Vasli et al. 2012). The latter application allows the sequencing of large genes such as *DMD* and *TTN* which are not routinely sequenced by the Sanger method. This type of analysis allowed the clinical spectrum of *TTN*-related diseases to be widened by noting a patient with myopathy with cytoplasmic aggregates and respiratory insufficiency widens the clinical spectrum compared to previous studies (Hackman et al. 2002).

A disadvantage of panel-based NGS approaches is that not all genes or gene regions associated with NMD are included either because of a target size limitation or a specific gene has yet to be associated with NMD. Vasli et al. failed to find the genetic cause for four patients with an unknown molecular diagnosis (Vasli et al. 2012). Patient I was first clinically diagnosed with demyelinating polyneuropathy, but clinical and biochemical reanalyses in parallel to NGS suggested he had a mitochondrial disease which implicated genes are not covered by this present design. Patient N showed two *in cis* missense changes in *LMNA* including the p.R644C change, previously linked to various laminopathies, and cannot explain the phenotype. Mutations were not identified in two patients by this NGS panel. Authors speculated that mutations may be deep intronic changes, repeat expansions, or translocation for which detection has not been tested in this study. Alternatively, patients may also be mutated in a gene not linked to NMD at the time of the targeting library design.

Whole exome sequencing or whole genome sequencing could potentially find the causative mutations and/or gene in patients without a molecular diagnosis and these must be added to the NMD capture library design. However, this WGS or WES has several disadvantages for routine molecular diagnosis compared to targeted panels. NMD-seq has a higher coverage and leads to a smaller list of variants as it focuses on a subset of genes, whereas the sensitivity and heterozygosity assessment decreases following WGS or WES due to lower coverage (Wheeler et al. 2008). Sequencing more genes at a lower coverage leads to an increased risk of false negative and an increased number of false positive variants that are time-consuming to validate. Therefore, the major reasons for use of the NMD panel strategy as a routine approach in genetic diagnostic laboratories are the reproducibility, detection sensitivity, and it applications to examine mutations in genetically heterogeneous disorders.

6.3 Next-Generation–Sequencing Panel for Duchenne and Becker, Congenital, and Limb Girdle Muscular Dystrophies

Duchenne muscular dystrophy and Becker muscular dystrophies are the most common forms of childhood muscular dystrophy (Emery 1991). Genetic testing of the *DMD* gene is commonly used to confirm the diagnosis. Defining the mutational spectrum is important for genetic counseling, prenatal diagnosis, and selecting the patients eligible for future mutation-specific treatments. The mutational spectrum can be approximated as follows: a large deletion in about 60 % of patients, a large duplication in about 10 % of patients, and small mutations confined mostly to coding exons in about 30 % of patients (Lim et al. 2011). In most laboratories, methods for detecting large deletions/duplications and methods for detecting small mutations are conducted separately (Bennett et al. 2001; Flanigan et al. 2003; Lalic et al. 2005; Mendell et al. 2001; Prior and Bridgeman 2005).

A study reports the application of NGS in the genetic diagnosis development of Duchenne muscular dystrophy or Becker and related muscular dystrophies to address diagnostic issues related to complex mutational spectrum, large size of the *DMD* gene, and the costly requirement of two or more analytical methods to account for known point, small indels, and large indel mutations (Table 6.1; Lim et al. 2011). The study subjects were 25 patients: 16 with deficient dystrophin expression without a large deletion/duplication and nine with a known large deletion/duplication. Technically, Lim et al. used a custom solution-based target enrichment kit for *DMD* and other muscular dystrophy-related genes and Illumina Genome Analyzer as a sequencing platform (Lim et al. 2011). The mean coverage of the *DMD* gene was 107X and exonic regions had at least the read depth of 8X. Significantly, small mutations were detected in most patients (15 out of 16) without a large deletion/duplication.

For the development of one platform for comprehensive *DMD* mutation analysis, Lim et al. used these 16 patients as the standard and accurately predicted the deleted or duplicated exons in the nine patients with known mutations. Pathogenic mutations were observed in 15 of 16 patients, and the mutation detection rate and distribution of mutation by types (12 nonsense, two small deletions causing frameshifts, and one splicing mutation) were similar to the results of other studies using different methods. Because 16 patients in this study were selected randomly and their genotypes were unconfirmed, the mutation detection rate might provide further support for the accuracy of this method. Additionally, inclusion of noncoding regions in the design permitted breakpoint junction mapping.

Lim et al. present a more practical approach by testing a relatively large number of patients and demonstrating the detection of complex mutational spectra in a single platform (Lim et al. 2011). This approach allows reaching a genetic diagnosis of DMD/BMD in a shorter time as compared to the combined MLPA and Sanger sequencing methods. Moreover, inclusion of other related genes might contribute to reduction of cost for clinical use. The current approach has an advantage for the genetic diagnosis of Duchenne muscular dystrophy and Becker muscular dystrophy wherein a comprehensive mutational search may be feasible using a single platform.

6.4   Duchenne and Becker Muscular Dystrophy Diagnosis by Next-Generation–Sequencing

Dystrophin is a large, rod-like cytoskeletal protein and located mainly in skeletal muscles and cardiac muscles (Xie et al. 2012). This protein stabilizes and protects muscle fibers and may play a role in signaling within cells. Mutations in the *DMD* gene can alter the structure or function of dystrophin resulting in fatal, X-linked disorder occurring at a frequency of about 1 in 3,500 new-born males (Sironi et al. 2006). There are two identified hot spots of *DMD* gene: the major hot spot involves the region of exons 40–55, while the minor one is located around intron 7 (Sironi et al. 2006). The high demand for low-cost and high-throughput sequencing has urged the development and progress of high-throughput NGS. With the need to obtain a genetic diagnosis more rapidly and to avoid the gene-by-gene Sanger sequencing approach, NGS' position on the stage of DNA sequencing and causative mutations detection is important (Sironi et al. 2006). To this end, a targeted NGS strategy was employed in detecting *DMD* gene mutations, a large gene containing 79 exons with different mutation types and regions (Xie et al. 2012).

Xie et al. carried out *DMD* mutation analysis by NGS, employing solid phase capture followed by HiSeq 2000 sequencing, on a Chinese pedigree that included a proband and a proband's cousin with the clinical diagnosis of Duchenne muscular dystrophy (Xie et al. 2012) (Table 6.1). The proband and proband's cousin developed symptoms of muscle weakness, difficulty walking, and large calves. Progressive muscle weakness resulted in the inability to walk, breathing difficulties, contractures of the ankles, knees, and hips, and scoliosis. For the *DMD* gene of the proband, the average depth was 471X, the average depth for each base pair was 160X, and the average median-depth across 79 exons was 168X. On average, 98.5 % of base pairs with greater than 20X coverage were successfully detected. Two same variants were detected in exon 70 of the proband and his cousin. A literature-annotated disease nonsense mutation (c.10141C>T, NM_004006.1) that has been reported as a *DMD* causing mutation was found in two patients, the proband and his cousin. Therefore, the nonsense led to the generation of a truncated dystrophin lacking the C-terminal domains. NGS was demonstrated to be an effective approach for determining the genetic cause and reaching a molecular diagnosis for the patients in the study.

6.5 Congenital Muscular Dystrophies Next-Generation– Sequencing Panel

Congenital muscular dystrophy disorders (CMD) can be classified into four major groups, based on the affected genes and the location of their expressed protein: (1) abnormalities of extracellular matrix proteins (*LAMA2*, *COL6A1*, *COL6A2*, and *COL6A3*); (2) abnormalities of membrane receptors for the extracellular matrix (*FKTN*, *POMGNT1*, *POMT1*, *POMT2*, *FKRP*, *LARGE*, *ITGA7*, and *DAG1*); (3) abnormal endoplasmic reticulum protein (*SEPN1*); and (4) intranuclear envelope protein (*LMNA*; Wang et al. 2010). A specific diagnosis can be challenging because muscle pathology may not yield a definitive diagnosis, limited access to and expertise in using immunohistochemical stains, and phenotypic as well as genetic heterogeneity. Muscle biopsy and genetic test findings must be interpreted in a clinical context, yet the majority of diagnostic testing is not accompanied by a standard clinical data set. Sequential gene sequencing by conventional Sanger sequencing has been routinely used to diagnose this group of muscular dystrophies even though it is a time-consuming and costly approach to resolve clinically heterogeneous genetic disorders.

Valencia et al. investigated the application of NGS technologies for the molecular diagnosis of CMD (Table 6.1; Valencia et al. 2012). To this end, the authors assessed the analytical sensitivity and specificity of two different enrichment technologies, solution-based hybridization (SS), and microdroplet multiplex PCR target enrichment (RainDance Technologies, RDT), in conjunction with NGS, to identify mutations in 321 exons representing 12 different genes (65 kb target region) involved with congenital muscular dystrophies (Valencia et al. 2012). In this study a wild-type control, which had all 12 CMD genes Sanger sequenced, was included to serve as a normal control reference, along with five positive control samples, with previously known mutations, blinded to laboratory staff and six blinded samples, with previously uncharacterized CMD genes, from patients presenting with clinical features of CMD.

Valencia et al. reported that NGS results across several parameters, including sequencing metrics and genotype concordance (Valencia et al. 2012). No statistically significant differences between the two enrichment methods were observed for average read numbers and percentage mapping to the genome. At 5X the coverage was 96 % and 88 % for SS and RDT samples, respectively. Unfortunately, regions with low sequence coverage typically had a high GC, making amplification difficult. Moreover, the genotype concordance of SS and RDT was less than

100 % when compared to Sanger sequencing due to the low coverage regions which is an inherent problem of the enrichment technologies and not the sequencing platform. However, in regions with greater than 20X read depth, the genotyping data showed that both enrichment technologies produced suitable calls for use in clinical laboratories.

Several parameters are worth comparing between the two enrichment technologies and contrasting them to Sanger sequencing; namely, clinical implementation, cost, requirement for specialized equipment, ease of use, analytical sensitivity and specificity, and scalability (Valencia et al. 2012). RDT offers the lowest enrichment cost per amplicon when compared to SS and Sanger sequencing. The RDT and SS DNA requirements are similar, but the Sanger method requires a significantly higher amount of DNA. RDT is more appropriate for situations requiring multiple genes with long exons because it can enrich a target interval up to 1 Mb. Up to eight samples can be processed per day. Similarly, SS can be used to process eight patients per day, but it can enrich a much larger target interval, up to the entire exome. By contrast, only one patient sample may be processed by Sanger sequencing in a day because it is such a large panel (383 amplicons). One important diagnostic issue is the ability to distinguish between gene and pseudogene targets; RDT and Sanger can readily address this issue by correctly choosing locations where the primers are to hybridize on the genomic DNA template. Since SS is a hybridization-based method, its limitation is not being able to distinguish between the gene and pseudogene targets. Therefore, RDT is more appropriate for a clinical laboratory, due to excellent sequence specificity and uniformity, reproducibility, high coverage of the target exons, and the ability to distinguish the active gene versus known pseudogenes. Regardless of the method, exons with highly repetitive and high GC regions are not well enriched and require Sanger sequencing for completeness. This study demonstrated the successful application of targeted sequencing in conjunction with NGS to screen for mutations in hundreds of exons in a genetically heterogeneous human disorder.

A recent study from the same group investigated the diagnostic yields from the implementation of the RDT CMD sequencing panel as compared to the single-gene Sanger sequencing approach (Valencia et al. 2013). Following a successful analytical validation, a clinical CMD NGS panel was launched at EGL and has been used successfully by clinicians in CMD cases presenting with overlapping phenotypes, inconclusive biochemical studies, and nondiagnostic brain or muscle MRIs. This expedited approach to molecular diagnosis avoids the diagnostic odyssey and cost associated with a serial gene testing approach. Valencia et al. demonstrated that the CMD panel approach convincingly showed better mutation detection or diagnostic yield compared to a single-gene analysis. The efficiency and better yield of the panel approach is better illustrated by the analysis of the 20 blinded samples included in the study. Several samples, which underwent a series of single-gene tests, and others which remained CMD of unknown molecular etiology due to inconclusive biochemical or immunologic assays, all received a definitive diagnosis through this NGS approach. Furthermore, the percent diagnostic yield of all EGL CMD tests and single-gene tests was 41 % and 17 %, respectively.

6.6   Summary

The NMD NGS panels offer cost-effective and more rapid molecular diagnostic testing than the conventional sequential Sanger sequencing of associated genes. A faster molecular diagnosis of NMD will have major impacts on patients as it will improve disease management and genetic counseling, and will allow access to therapy or inclusion into therapeutic trials. However, the targeted sequencing strategy has limitations. As the current methods did not equal Sanger sequencing in terms of analytical sensitivity and specificity, mainly because of insufficient coverage of target regions, complementary Sanger sequencing seems to be necessary. Furthermore, for the application of this approach to be used in clinical molecular diagnostics, the analytical sensitivity and specificity need to be determined according to the individualized target enrichment methods and sequencing platforms.

References

Bennett RR, den Dunnen J, O'Brien KF et al (2001) Detection of mutations in the dystrophin gene via automated DHPLC screening and direct sequencing. BMC Genet 2:17

Emery AE (1991) Population frequencies of inherited neuromuscular diseases—a world survey. Neuromuscul Disord 1:19–29

Flanigan KM, von Niederhausern A, Dunn DM et al (2003) Rapid direct sequence analysis of the dystrophin gene. Am J Hum Genet 72:931–939

Hackman P, Vihola A, Haravuori H et al (2002) Tibial muscular dystrophy is a titinopathy caused by mutations in TTN, the gene encoding the giant skeletal-muscle protein titin. Am J Hum Genet 71:492–500. doi:10.1086/342380

Lalic T, Vossen RHAM, Coffa J et al (2005) Deletion and duplication screening in the DMD gene using MLPA. Eur J Hum Genet 13:1231–1234. doi:10.1038/sj.ejhg.5201465

Lim BC, Lee S, Shin J-Y et al (2011) Genetic diagnosis of Duchenne and Becker muscular dystrophy using next-generation sequencing technology: comprehensive mutational search in a single platform. J Med Genet 48:731–736. doi:10.1136/jmedgenet-2011-100133

Mendell JR, Buzin CH, Feng J et al (2001) Diagnosis of Duchenne dystrophy by enhanced detection of small mutations. Neurology 57:645–650

North K (2008) What's new in congenital myopathies? Neuromuscul Disord 18:433–442. doi:10.1016/j.nmd.2008.04.002

Prior TW, Bridgeman SJ (2005) Experience and strategy for the molecular testing of Duchenne muscular dystrophy. J Mol Diagn 7:317–326. doi:10.1016/S1525-1578(10)60560-0

Sironi M, Pozzoli U, Comi GP et al (2006) A region in the dystrophin gene major hot spot harbors a cluster of deletion breakpoints and generates double-strand breaks in yeast. FASEB J 20:1910–1912. doi:10.1096/fj.05-5635fje

Valencia CA, Rhodenizer D, Bhide S et al (2012) Assessment of target enrichment platforms using massively parallel sequencing for the mutation detection for congenital muscular dystrophy. J Mol Diagn 14:233–246. doi:10.1016/j.jmoldx.2012.01.009

Valencia CA, Ankala A, Rhodenizer D et al (2013) Comprehensive mutation analysis for congenital muscular dystrophy: a clinical PCR-based enrichment and next-generation sequencing panel. PLoS One 8:e53083. doi:10.1371/journal.pone.0053083

Vasli N, Böhm J, Le Gras S et al (2012) Next-generation sequencing for molecular diagnosis of neuromuscular diseases. Acta Neuropathol (Berl) 124:273–283. doi:10.1007/s00401-012-0982-8

Wang CH, Bonnemann CG, Rutkowski A et al (2010) Consensus statement on standard of care for congenital muscular dystrophies. J Child Neurol 25:1559–1581. doi:10.1177/0883073810381924

Wheeler DA, Srinivasan M, Egholm M et al (2008) The complete genome of an individual by massively parallel DNA sequencing. Nature 452:872–876. doi:10.1038/nature06884

Xie S, Lan Z, Qu N et al (2012) Detection of truncated dystrophin lacking the C-terminal domain in a Chinese pedigree by next-generation sequencing. Gene 499:139–142. doi:10.1016/j.gene.2012.03.029

Chapter 7
Application of Next-Generation–Sequencing in Hearing Loss Diagnosis

7.1 Introduction

Hearing loss is the most common birth defect and sensorineural disorder in humans. Hearing loss results from obstructions in the transmission of the sound anywhere between the outer ear and auditory cortex in the brain. In a normal condition, the sound signal that is collected by the outer ear is amplified by the middle ear for transmission to the cochlea, which then converts this energy into electrical signals that are ultimately transmitted to the brain through the auditory nerves (Smith et al. 1993). Based on the defective anatomical structure involved, hearing loss can be classified as conductive, sensorineural, or mixed. Conductive hearing loss is a defect in conducting sound waves through outer and middle ear due to abnormalities of outer ear, tympanic membrane (eardrum), or ossicles of the middle ear. Sensorineural hearing loss (SNHL) is due to a defect located anywhere from cochlea to the auditory cortex. Mixed hearing loss is a combination of both conductive and sensorineural abnormalities. Depending on the age at onset, hearing loss can be classified as prelingual, present before speech development, or postlingual, present after speech development. Severity of the hearing loss is measured by decibels (dB), can be graded from mild (26–40 dB) to profound (90 dB), affecting from low to high frequencies (Smith et al. 1993).

In this chapter, we introduce syndromic and nonsyndromic hearing loss (NSHL) alongside the importance of hearing loss detection. Then, we focus on covering the recent advances of hearing loss diagnosis in light of the application of next-generation–sequencing (NGS) to this field.

7.2 Hearing Loss Syndromes

One in 500 newborns is affected with bilateral permanent SNHL in developed countries; this number is increased to 2.7 per 1,000 before the age of 5 years and 3.5 per 1,000 during adolescence (Morton and Nance 2006). Approximately two-thirds of

C.A. Valencia et al., *Next Generation Sequencing Technologies in Medical Genetics*, SpringerBriefs in Genetics, DOI 10.1007/978-1-4614-9032-6_7, hearing loss is due to genetic factors and, in the remaining one-third of cases, it is caused by environmental factors (Hilgert et al. 2009; Raviv et al. 2010). The environmental factors that cause hearing loss include both prenatal and postnatal infections, use of ototoxic drugs, and exposure to excessive noise. The majority of the inherited form of hearing loss is monogenic, and it can be syndromic or nonsyndromic. In the syndromic forms, hearing loss is accompanied by other physical manifestations, and it accounts for about 30 % of the inherited hearing loss (Kochhar et al. 2007). Over 400 syndromes have been reported with hearing loss, and some of the common forms of syndromic hearing loss including Usher, Pendred, Jervell and Lange-Nielsen, Waardenburg, Branchio-oto-renal, and Stickler syndromes are among the many (Cohen and Phillips 2012; Hilgert et al. 2009). The nonsyndromic forms of hearing loss, with no other physical findings, account for about 70 % of inherited hearing loss. They are categorized into four different groups according to their mode of inheritance: (1) autosomal recessive, (2) autosomal dominant, (3) X-linked, and (4) maternal inheritance due to mutations in mitochondrial genes. The autosomal recessive hearing loss is the most common type occurring in about 80 % of patients, followed by autosomal dominant in about 20 %. The X-linked and mitochondrial hearing loss are less common and account for only about 1 % of the patients (Brownstein and Avraham 2009; Van Camp et al. 1997; Vandebona et al. 2009).

7.3 Nonsyndromic Hearing Loss

NSHL is extremely heterogeneous and, so far, over 150 loci responsible for this form of hearing loss have been mapped. These loci are designated as DFN that is derived from abbreviation of *DeaFN*ess followed by mode of transmission; DFNA refers to loci for autosomal dominant forms, DFNB refers to loci for autosomal recessive, and DFNX to X-linked forms. The numbers following the designation are chronological order of locus identification (DFNB1 refers to first autosomal recessive locus). To date, 40 autosomal recessive (ARNSHL), 27 autosomal dominant (ADNSHL), three X-linked, and two mitochondrial genes have been identified. Many of these genes cause more than one form of hearing loss. For example, *SLC26A4*, *CDH23*, *MYO7A*, *DFNB31*, *USH1C*, and others cause both syndromic and nonsyndromic forms; *TMC1*, *GJB2*, *GJB6*, *MYO7A*, and others may cause both autosomal dominant and autosomal recessive forms of hearing loss. Mutations in the *GJB2*, encoding connexin 26, that cause DFNB1 are the most common cause of hearing loss and account for about 50 % of the cases with autosomal recessive hearing loss in many populations (Cohen and Phillips 2012; Kochhar et al. 2007). The remaining cases are attributable to the mutations in other genes, and among others *SLC26A4*, *MYO7A*, *OTOF*, *CDH23*, and *TMC1* are more prevalent (Hilgert et al. 2009). Mutations in the rest of the genes are very rare; many of them have been found to cause hearing loss in one or two consanguineous families (Kochhar et al. 2007; Zbar et al. 1998). Except *WFS1*, *KCNQ4*, *GJB2*, and *COCH*, most of the genes causing autosomal dominant hearing loss are not a common cause of hearing loss (Hilgert et al. 2009).

7.4 Importance of Hearing Loss Detection and Genetic Testing

Early detection and intervention for children with hearing loss offers opportunities for improving language and speech development, thereby facilitating the acquisition of normal social and cognitive skills. Elucidation of the genetic basis of hearing loss is crucial for the clinical management of patients and their family. In addition, determination of genetic etiology in a large cohort of patients will provide better understanding of genotype–phenotype correlations, which could help developing specific therapeutic interventions. For syndromic hearing loss, selection of causative genes to reach a molecular diagnosis are possible based on associated symptoms, whereas this approach is not feasible for nonsyndromic hearing loss because phenotype caused by most of the genes is indistinguishable. Therefore, sequential screening of all hearing loss genes has been widely applied to identify the genetic cause. Currently, genetic testing for hearing loss is conducted using different diagnostic algorithms in several institutions worldwide. Mutation screening of coding and flanking intronic regions of the candidate genes using automated Sanger sequencing is the most common approach in vast the majority of these laboratories. However, the extreme genetic heterogeneity of nonsyndromic and syndromic hearing loss makes this strategy unfavorable in terms of cost and time. NGS technology offers the advantage of sequencing multiple genes in parallel with lower cost and higher time-efficiency.

7.5 Capture-Based Hearing Loss Panels

Shearer et al. developed a comprehensive diagnostic platform named as OtoSCOPE that targeted the exons of 54 known NSHL genes including Usher syndrome genes (Table 7.1; Shearer et al. 2010). In this study, two hybridization capture-based enrichment approaches, NimbleGen solid-phase enrichment and Agilent SureSelect (SS) solution-based capture enrichment, were paired with 454 GS FLX pyrosequencing and Illumina GAII cyclic reversible termination sequencing, respectively. By comparing these two platforms, SS-Illumina was shown to be superior in terms of scalability, cost, and increased sensitivity, generating a 13-fold higher average depth of coverage on targeted bases (903x vs 71x), with 95.3 % of targeted hearing loss genes covered at 40x threshold (Table 7.1). Highly heterozygous SNPs in the target regions were confirmed by Sanger sequencing to determine the sensitivity and specificity, which were both greater than 99 % for the SS-Illumina platform. Besides the use of three patients as positive controls, NSHL mutations were found in *STRC*, *MYO6*, *KCNQ4*, *MYN14*, and *CDH23* genes in five out of six idiopathic SNHL patients, including three novel mutations. However, the variants found in one patient were ruled out as causative mutations by segregation analysis. Similarly, a capture-based enrichment approach was used in another study that was designed to

Table 7.1 Performance of next-generation–sequencing platforms for mutation detection of hearing loss genes

	Capture-based HL gene panel			PCR-based HL gene panel				Whole exome sequencing		
Target	54 known HL genes in human	54 known HL genes in human	246 known HL genes in human and mouse	15 known HL genes in human	34 known HL genes in human	24 known HL genes in human	9 known USH genes in human	Human Exome	Human Exome	Human Exome
Target enrichment method	NimbleGen solid-based enrichment	Agilent SureSelect solution-based enrichment	Agilent SureSelect solution-based enrichment	PCR-based amplification enrichment	RDT microdroplet PCR enrichment	RDT microdroplet PCR enrichment	Long-PCR enrichment	Agilent SureSelect 50 Mb enrichment	Illumina TrueSeq 62 Mb enrichment	Agilent SureSelect 50 Mb enrichment
Sequencing platform	Roche 454 GS FLX	Illumina GAII	Illumina GAII	Roche 454 GS FLX	Illumina HiSeq 2000	Illumina HiSeq 2000	Roche 454 GS FLX and Illumina GAII	Illumina HiSeq 2000	Illumina HiSeq 2000	SOLiD 3 or 4 Systems
Mean target coverage	71x	903x	757x	~150x	1,585x	NA	NA	NA	NA	NA
%Target coverage at calling threshold	96 %	95.30 %	95 %	95 %	95 %	96 %	94 %	57 %	65 %	~50 %
Minimum calling threshold	3x	40x	10x	30x	30x	40x	25x	20x	20x	25x
Sensitivity	93.98 %	99.72 %	NA	NA	99.00 %	>99.99 %	NA	NA	NA	NA
Specificity	97.92 %	>99.00 %	NA	NA	99.40 %	>99.99 %	NA	NA	NA	NA
References	Shearer et al. (2010)	Shearer et al. (2010)	Brownstein et al. (2011)	De Keulenaer et al. (2012)	Schrauwen et al. (2013)	Sivakumaran et al. (2013)	Licastro et al. (2012)	Schrauwen et al. (2013)	Schrauwen et al. (2013)	Licastro et al. (2012)

HL hearing loss, *RDT* RainDance Technologies, *NA* not available detect 246 genes responsible for either human or mouse deafness. With a 95 % of coverage of the targeted bases at 10x, pathogenic mutations were identified in six of the 11 probands and their families in *CDH23, MYO15A, TECTA, TMC1*, and *WFS1* (Brownstein et al. 2011).

Even though successes have been shown, hybridization capture-based enrichment has restrictions in the capture of GC-rich or repetitive elements as well as gene family members that share sequence homology. The presence of repetitive or high GC content sequences results in incomplete selection, selection bias, and uneven capture efficiency. This may result in reduced sensitivity and specificity that are highly required in diagnostic testing (De Keulenaer et al. 2012; Schrauwen et al. 2013). To address these disadvantages, PCR amplification-based enrichment has been employed in several hearing loss studies followed by NGS.

7.5.1   PCR-Based Hearing Loss Panels

A European group designed a primer library including 646 specific primer pairs for exons and most of the UTR of 15 ARNSHL genes, using semiautomated conventional PCR. All amplicons were pooled in an equal molar concentration and analyzed using Roche 454 NGS technology (Table 7.1; De Keulenaer et al. 2012). This platform generated the coverage of 95 % targeted bases at 30x depth. Among five patients with congenital genetic deafness, causative mutations were identified in four patients. Among these, two novel mutations in *CDH23* and *OTOF* were found in three patients that were also characterized as interesting regions in a previous linkage study. Similarly, Licastro et al. used a long-PCR-based enrichment and NGS to develop a diagnostic panel for Usher syndrome genes (Licastro et al. 2012). Molecular diagnosis in Usher syndrome is hindered by significant genetic heterogeneity, the large size of some of the Usher genes, numerous polymorphic variants in genes such as *MYO7A* and *USH2A*, and digenic inheritance which was also proposed in some Usher syndrome cases (Bonnet et al. 2011). At least 11 loci and nine causative genes have been reported associated with three subtypes of Usher syndrome. Current diagnostic strategies for Usher syndrome include Sanger sequencing of Usher genes, which is a demanding procedure in terms of both cost and time, or microarrays-based genotyping method that only detects the previously reported mutation. This study showed this NGS platform had 94 % coverage of target bases at 25x. Eleven pathogenic mutations in *MYO7A, CLRN1, GPR98, USH2A*, and *PCDH15* were identified in ten out of the 12 USHER patients, while genetic causation of two patients still stayed negative, indicating a positive diagnostic rate of 84 % in this study.

The main advantage of microdroplet PCR-based technology, such as RainDance, is able to combine high-throughput automation and highly sensitive, specific, and uniform amplification using target specific primers (Tewhey et al. 2009). Recently, two research groups used a similar strategy, applying RDT microdroplet PCR enrichment and sequencing on the Illumina HiSeq 2000 sequencer, to develop NGS hearing loss panels for 34 ARNSHL genes and 24 well-studied SNHL genes, respectively (Schrauwen et al. 2013; Sivakumaran et al. 2013). The two NGS platforms targeted all exons and flanking intron regions of the hearing loss genes. Schrauwen et al. presented an overall mean coverage depth in the target area of 1,585x and 95 % of the bases were covered at 30x, while the panel developed by Sivakumaran et al. had a 96 % of the targeted bases covered at 40x. Sanger sequencing was used to verify the known variants. These two NGS panels both achieved >99 % sensitivity and specificity, indicating that the enrichment is a reliable platform for mutation detection of hearing loss genes.

To detect the concordance between NGS panel and Sanger sequencing, Sivakumaran et al. used the NextGENe software (SoftGenetics, LLC) which detected a total of 394 variants in five genes, *GJB2*, *CDH23*, *MYO7A*, *EYA1*, and *OTOF*, that had been sequenced by Sanger sequencing to confirm the accuracy. The results showed a >99.99 % concordance between NGS and Sanger sequencing by evaluating more than 30,000 bp in the five SNHL genes, except that only one C>T substitution in *MYO7A* detected by NGS was not identified by Sanger sequencing due to a misalignment issue. Small indels were detected in the NGS data including a 22-bp deletion in intron 27 of *MYO7A*. Since the acceptable false-positive and false-negative rates are more stringent for clinical diagnostic use, the authors favorably suggested to set >40x as coverage threshold at the target bases (Sivakumaran et al. 2013).

In the panel Schrauwen et al. designed, all genes were selected from an ARNSHL gene list and 24 patients with prelingual, moderate to profound hereditary NSHL in autosomal recessive inheritance, and without *GJB2* mutations were carefully selected. Nine out of 24 patients (37.5 %) were confidently diagnosed. Six patients were found to have homozygous mutations and three patients had compound heterozygous mutations. The results also suggested a possible digenic finding in *OTOF* and *SLC26A4* genes in one patient. However, these two genes perform completely different functions in the inner ear and proteins are expressed at different ear locations which weakened the evidence of digenic inheritance in this patient. The convincing follow-up family study is an important step to confirm the diagnosis (Schrauwen et al. 2013).

7.6   Whole Exome Sequencing

Whole exome sequencing is emerging as a diagnostic tool for many inherited diseases (Table 7.1; Chap. 8; Licastro et al. 2012; Schrauwen et al. 2013). However, comparison between the performance of RDT deafness libraries to the Agilent SureSelect 50 Mb Exome, Illumina TrueSeq 62 Mb exome, and Agilent SureSelect exome kits only had 50–67 % of the targeted deafness gene exons covered at 20x (Table 7.1). These results suggest that current exome sequencing does not provide sufficient target enrichment for hearing loss genes. However, improvement in capture technologies may increase the coverage in the near future.

7.7 Summary

NGS platforms provide a great potential that can lower cost by increasing capacity without compromising diagnostic standards. It becomes possible to screen a large number of known deafness genes, by the implementation of NGS technologies, at a price that would only allow a few genes to be analyzed by Sanger sequencing. This inclusion of more genes to panels has also made it possible to detect novel mutations in genes that were rarely tested, thus, expanding the list of mutations-associated hearing loss. Technically, comparisons of NGS platforms developed for hearing loss illustrated that microdroplet PCR-based enrichment exhibited overall superior standards and appeared to be a more promising technology in terms of a combination of high sensitivity, speed, and cost efficiency, and is reliable for clinical diagnosis, even though hybridization-based capture enrichment has the advantage of reducing the cost and workload. Application of NGS in clinical laboratories will greatly improve the diagnostic rate of hearing loss, and improve earlier intervention in patients with hearing loss. Subsequently, earlier implementation of educational services and medical treatment will positively change the life quality of the patients.

References

Bonnet C, Grati M, Marlin S et al (2011) Complete exon sequencing of all known Usher syndrome genes greatly improves molecular diagnosis. Orphanet J Rare Dis 6:21. doi:10.1186/1750-1172-6-21

Brownstein Z, Avraham KB (2009) Deafness genes in Israel: implications for diagnostics in the clinic. Pediatr Res 66:128–134. doi:10.1203/PDR.0b013e3181aabd7f

Brownstein Z, Friedman LM, Shahin H et al (2011) Targeted genomic capture and massively parallel sequencing to identify genes for hereditary hearing loss in Middle Eastern families. Genome Biol 12:R89. doi:10.1186/gb-2011-12-9-r89

Cohen M, Phillips JA 3rd (2012) Genetic approach to evaluation of hearing loss. Otolaryngol Clin North Am 45:25–39. doi:10.1016/j.otc.2011.08.015

De Keulenaer S, Hellemans J, Lefever S et al (2012) Molecular diagnostics for congenital hearing loss including 15 deafness genes using a next-generation sequencing platform. BMC Med Genomics 5:17. doi:10.1186/1755-8794-5-17

Hilgert N, Smith RJH, Van Camp G (2009) Forty-six genes causing nonsyndromic hearing impairment: which ones should be analyzed in DNA diagnostics? Mutat Res 681:189–196. doi:10.1016/j.mrrev.2008.08.002

Kochhar A, Hildebrand MS, Smith RJH (2007) Clinical aspects of hereditary hearing loss. Genet Med 9:393–408. doi:10.1097/GIM.0b013e3180980bd0

Licastro D, Mutarelli M, Peluso I et al (2012) Molecular diagnosis of Usher syndrome: application of two different next-generation sequencing-based procedures. PLoS One 7:e43799. doi:10.1371/journal.pone.0043799

Morton CC, Nance WE (2006) Newborn hearing screening—a silent revolution. N Engl J Med 354:2151–2164. doi:10.1056/NEJMra050700

Raviv D, Dror AA, Avraham KB (2010) Hearing loss: a common disorder caused by many rare alleles. Ann N Y Acad Sci 1214:168–179. doi:10.1111/j.1749-6632.2010.05868.x

Schrauwen I, Sommen M, Corneveaux JJ et al (2013) A sensitive and specific diagnostic test for hearing loss using a microdroplet PCR-based approach and next-generation sequencing. Am J Med Genet A 161:145–152. doi:10.1002/ajmg.a.35737

Shearer AE, DeLuca AP, Hildebrand MS et al (2010) Comprehensive genetic testing for hereditary hearing loss using massively parallel sequencing. Proc Natl Acad Sci U S A 107:21104–21109. doi:10.1073/pnas.1012989107

Sivakumaran TA, Husami A, Kissell D et al (2013) Performance evaluation of the next-generation sequencing approach for molecular diagnosis of hereditary hearing loss. Otolaryngol Head Neck Surg. doi:10.1177/0194599813482294

Smith RJ, Shearer AE, Hildebrand MS, Van Camp G (1993) Deafness and hereditary hearing loss overview. GeneReviews™

Tewhey R, Warner JB, Nakano M et al (2009) Microdroplet-based PCR enrichment for large-scale targeted sequencing. Nat Biotechnol 27:1025–1031. doi:10.1038/nbt.1583

Van Camp G, Willems PJ, Smith RJ (1997) Nonsyndromic hearing impairment: unparalleled heterogeneity. Am J Hum Genet 60:758–764

Vandebona H, Mitchell P, Manwaring N et al (2009) Prevalence of mitochondrial 1555A→G mutation in adults of European descent. N Engl J Med 360:642–644. doi:10.1056/NEJMc0806397

Voelkerding KV, Dames S, Durtschi JD (2010) Next-generation sequencing for clinical diagnostics—principles and application to targeted resequencing for hypertrophic cardiomyopathy: a paper from the 2009 William Beaumont Hospital Symposium on Molecular Pathology. J Mol Diagn 12:539–551. doi:10.2353/jmoldx.2010.100043

Zbar RI, Ramesh A, Srisailapathy CR et al (1998) Passage to India: the search for genes causing autosomal recessive nonsyndromic hearing loss. Otolaryngol Head Neck Surg 118:333–337

Chapter 8
Exome Sequencing as a Discovery and Diagnostic Tool

8.1 Introduction

The estimated size of the human genome is 2,872 Mbps consisting of genes and noncoding sequences of DNA. Approximately 1.5 % of the human genome is known to code for proteins and this portion is the exome. This coding portion has been shown to be more evolutionary-conserved, thus more sensitive to change (Birney et al. 2007). The decreasing cost of sequencing, due to emerging next-generation–sequencing (NGS) technologies, provides an opportunity to screen the exome at an affordable cost for gene discovery and diagnostic purposes. The great amount of information generated from the human genome sequencing, 1000 genomes project, HapMap, and whole exome sequencing (WES) projects has allowed us to interpret sequence changes with a higher level of confidence (Abecasis et al. 2012, 2010; Tennessen et al. 2012). To deal with the large sequencing datasets, a variety of bio-informatics tools have been developed to automate the process of annotation and prediction of sequence changes (Wang et al. 2010b). Due to the massive parallel nature of NGS, research and clinical applications of NGS include the sequencing of many genes, as targeted panels, exomes, and even genomes. An increase in published findings has allowed cataloging of polymorphisms and disease-associated mutations at various databases that include the database of single nucleotide polymorphisms (dbSNP), the human gene mutation database (HGMD), ENSEMBL, the 1000 genomes project database (http://www.1000genomes.org/), and the exome sequencing project database (http://evs.gs.washington.edu/EVS/) to mention a few. The large data is evident in dbSNP that has close to 53 million records and the number of new submissions has been exponentially increasing (Wheeler et al. 2007).

For the past 5 years WES has been used successfully applied as a diagnostic tool, in the clinical area, and as a discovery tool to find new disease genes (Bolze et al. 2010; Coelho et al. 2012; Dibbens et al. 2013; Yu et al. 2013). In these studies, family-based analysis designs provide a simple means of cross sample hypothesis testing (Ku et al. 2011). About 180,000 exons are targeted for array or solution-based capture methods followed by NGS (Okou et al. 2007; Sulonen et al. 2011).

C.A. Valencia et al., *Next Generation Sequencing Technologies in Medical Genetics*,
SpringerBriefs in Genetics, DOI 10.1007/978-1-4614-9032-6_8,
© C. Alexander Valencia 2013

While family-based analysis designs allow for disease gene discoveries, the data from these efforts provides the name of the gene and better molecular description of the human exome by contributing to the frequency information of known and novel SNPs. In addition, the increase in sequencing data output (depth of coverage) has increased the sequencing accuracy and improvement of exome enrichment methods has opened the opportunity to use the exome as a clinical diagnostic tool and the clinical exome test is now being offered by several clinical laboratories. To continue the data curation, bioinformatic procedures include reduction or correction of sequencing errors by intra- and inter-sample comparisons.

A major challenge in WES is narrowing down the number of variants to a manageable potentially causative gene list. The exome analysis pipeline can be used in research to discover new genes associated with disease as well as its clinical application to medical genetics. Previous chapters have covered the sequencing (Chap. 2) and enrichment technologies (Chap. 3) in depth; thus, the focus here is to summarize the reported applications of WES to research and the molecular diagnostic fields. In addition, we briefly describe the bioinformatic procedures that are performed to identify the potential causative genes and tools used in the interpretation of variants.

8.2 Classic Gene Discovery Approaches and Limitations

In the past, traditional linkage studies have been used to identify causal variants or mutation for Mendelian (single gene or monogenic) disorders (Botstein and Risch 2003). Examples of Mendelian disorders include Freeman–Sheldon syndrome, Fowler syndrome, autosomal-dominant amyotrophic lateral sclerosis, and hypercholesterolemia (Ng et al. 2009; Lalonde et al. 2010; Johnson et al. 2010a; Rios et al. 2010). Thus far, causal variants for approximately 3,000 Mendelian disorders have been discovered and are cataloged by the Online Mendelian Inheritance in Man (OMIM; http://www.ncbi.nlm.nih.gov/omim).

Due to the perfect segregation (high penetrance), genome-wide linkage studies followed by positional cloning have also identified causal variants of Mendelian disorders. In principle, genome-wide linkage studies assume no prior hypothesis because the genetic markers will evenly cover the whole genome. Only a limited number of recombination events are observed within a family or pedigree. The genetic markers will reveal genomic regions which co-segregated in affected individuals. This could then be followed up by positional cloning to identify the causal variants and candidate genes within the genomic regions, which can be up to tens of centimorgans (cM). On the contrary, candidate gene-based linkage studies require a prior hypothesis and are not designed to reveal novel genomic regions for Mendelian disorders (Botstein and Risch 2003).

Classical linkage studies have been the main approach for discovering causal variants of Mendelian disorders; however, not all of these disorders are amendable to this study design. Homozygosity mapping, on the other hand, is a more powerful and effective approach to study recessive disorders in consanguineous families (Harville et al. 2010; Collin et al. 2010; Pang et al. 2010; Iseri et al. 2010). However, the causal variants remain elusive for many disorders that cannot use these two approaches. These disorders include (1) "extremely rare" Mendelian disorders, where only a small number of cases are available, (2) unrelated cases from different families, and (3) sporadic cases due to de novo variants (Ku et al. 2011). However, WES now offers new opportunities to study extremely rare disorders and sporadic cases as well as complex diseases.

8.3   Exome Sequencing Necessity for Gene Discovery

The linkage study design is unsuitable for the de novo variants and extremely rare Mendelian disorders because of the difficulty in collection of an adequate number of affected individuals (of multigenerational pedigree) and families for a statistically powerful study (Ku et al. 2011). For example, the candidate gene for Kabuki syndrome remained unknown until recently because it is an extremely rare (incidence 1 in 32,000) autosomal-dominant Mendelian disorder (Ng et al. 2010a). To address these issues, WES was performed on ten individuals affected with Kabuki syndrome and causal variants were found in *MLL2* (Ng et al. 2010a). Similarly, Schinzel–Giedion syndrome cases are mostly sporadic. Through WES de novo causal variants were identified in *SETBP1* in four affected individuals with this syndrome (Hoischen et al. 2010). Moreover, the causative variants of Miller syndrome, an extremely rare disorder, were recently reported in *DHODH* (Ng et al. 2010b). Collectively, these studies have demonstrated the advantages of WES over the linkage study design in situations where a small number of unrelated samples or sporadic cases are available.

In contrast to linkage study designs, WES is more robust for disorders with presumably genetic and phenotypic heterogeneity (Ku et al. 2011). These problems are well depicted in Kabuki syndrome which is likely a genetically heterogeneous disorder because not all the affected individuals have causal variants in the single candidate gene (*MLL2*; Ng et al. 2010a). However, causal variants in other genes have not been identified. By accounting for the genetic and phenotypic heterogeneity, the investigators successfully identified causal variants in *MLL2* in a subset of individuals. WES has now become technically feasible and more cost-effective due to the recent advances in high-throughput sequence capture methods and NGS technologies, which have offered new opportunities for Mendelian disorder research.

8.4   Exome Sequencing Gene Discovery Applications

8.4.1   Sequencing of Unrelated Individuals

The WES approach has been clearly demonstrated to be useful for identification of causative variants of extremely rare Mendelian disorders, especially for de novo variants that were not addressed by linkage studies, by sequencing the exomes of unrelated affected individuals. For example, four unrelated cases were subjected to WES and *MYH3* was identified as the single candidate gene for Freeman–Sheldon syndrome with variants that had not been previously reported in dbSNP and HapMap databases (Ng et al. 2009). A similar strategy was used by the same group to identify the candidate gene for Kabuki syndrome (Ng et al. 2010a). Specifically, the exomes of ten unrelated individuals affected with Kabuki syndrome were sequenced. However, to account for genetic heterogeneity, a less stringent strategy was applied by performing a search of the candidate genes shared among subsets of affected individuals. Additionally, various ranking and stratifying steps were also taken to account for phenotypic heterogeneity. These additional strategies finally led to the identification of causal variants in the *MLL2* gene. The *MLL2* gene of 43 of affected individuals was screened by Sanger sequencing. Interestingly, 12 individuals had de novo variants. Similarly, only two out of eight individuals with Sensenbrenner syndrome had causal variants in *WDR35* (Gilissen et al. 2010). These causal variants were only identified in two unrelated cases with a strikingly similar phenotype. This highlights the complexity of genetic and phenotypic heterogeneity and implies that classifying phenotypic heterogeneity helps in identifying the causal variants. Further studies have also identified a number of novel candidate genes harboring causal variants for disorders such as Miller syndrome, Fowler syndrome, Perrault syndrome, and Schinzel–Giedion syndrome (Ng et al. 2010b; Hoischen et al. 2010; Lalonde et al. 2010; Pierce et al. 2010). These studies show the feasibility of applying WES to identify the candidate genes for Mendelian disorders using unrelated cases. Furthermore, other studies have applied a combination of WES strategies to identify candidate genes, namely, WES with linkage or homozygosity analysis.

8.4.2 Sequencing of Family Members

Reported WES strategies have included performing analysis on affected individuals within a family. Autosomal-dominant spinocerebellar ataxias, previously studied disorders, have been examined by WES to identify new candidate genes (Ku et al. 2011). To date, causal variants in 20 genes have been identified for this disorder (Wang et al. 2010a). Authors performed WES in four affected individuals in one four-generation Chinese family with autosomal-dominant spinocerebellar ataxias. One of the advantages of this strategy is that it allowed investigators to hypothesize that all affected individuals should share the same causal variant, as spinocerebellar ataxia was inherited in an autosomal-dominant pattern in this family, which was supported by linkage analysis. Spinocerebellar ataxias are also characterized by clinical and genetic heterogeneity which would benefit from WES. The sequencing of affected individuals in one family would offer further advantage to the study design as unrelated cases from different families are likely to have causal variants in different genes. Other studies have also performed WES in multiple siblings and identified causal variants and candidate genes for disorders such as autosomal-dominant amyotrophic lateral sclerosis, familial combined hypolipidemia, and hyperphosphatasia mental retardation syndrome (Krawitz et al. 2010; Musunuru et al. 2010; Johnson et al. 2010b). In addition, WES has also been swiftly integrated with homozygosity mapping to accelerate the investigation of recessive disorders in consanguineous families (Walsh et al. 2010; Bolze et al. 2010).

8.4.3 Implementation of Family-Based Analysis as a Discovery Tool

Tens of thousands of single nucleotide variants and short indels are detected in the sequencing of the human exome and multiple filtering criteria are typically employed for the identification of causal variants. These filters include inheritance models, frequency, mutation types (nonsynonymous variants, splice-site disruptions, or coding indels), predictions, functional classification, and literature findings, to mention a few. As shown in the previous sections, these filters have proven effective in identifying candidate genes for several Mendelian disorders and the filtering process, which is the essence of exome analysis, will be discussed below.

8.4.3.1 Primary, Secondary, and Tertiary Variant Filtering

The general workflow of NGS variant detection analysis is summarized in three major phases. The primary phase is the process of generating base calls combined with quality control filtering, which is performed automatically after the image acquisition (Illumina HiSeq2000/MiSeq, Roche/454 Genome Sequencer) on the instrument-attached computer, and generates FASTQ files for the second step (Fig. 8.1). The throughput depends on the instrument, typically producing 30–45,000 variants per exome on 100 paired-end cycles.

The secondary phase is the process of alignment to the human genome reference sequence combined with quality filtering to remove common sequencing errors (Fig. 8.1). Typically, 98 % of the high quality reads are expected to align to the human genome reference sequence (Genome Reference Consortium, GRCh37). Directly after the alignment, a process of determining variants by comparison of consensus to genome reference is performed. This process of variant detection is followed by an annotation step where gene features, such as functional predictions, conservation, and others, are added to each variant. Example of commercial software that perform thousands of variant annotations per hour is Alamut-HT and adds the information from other databases such as dbSNP, OMIM, and HGMD and provides precomputed predictions for various prediction tools, like and ANNOVAR. Examples of prediction tools that are publicly available are PANTHER (Protein Analysis Through Evolutionary Relationships), SIFT (Sorting Intolerant From Tolerant amino acid substitutions), and Polyphen-2.

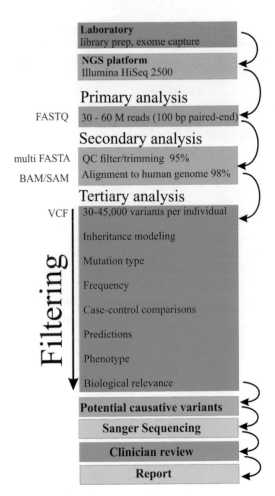

Fig. 8.1 Whole exome sequencing workflow. The DNA is fragmented, library is prepared, and reads are generated by NGS instrument (i.e., HiSeq2500). Determining nucleotide calls (A,C,G,T or N) along with error probabilities (Q score) is performed via a proprietary base calling algorithm during the sequencing run. The FASTQ file is the raw data which contains the base calls and quality score per base. The major step in the analysis is the process of aligning the reads to the human genome, which often takes few hours to complete. To assess the quality of exome sequencing QC parameters, which include the number of reads aligned successfully and the depth of coverage percentage on specific target region, are checked. The alignment procedure yields multi-sequence alignments in BAM format. Next, variants are determined by comparison to an indexed reference sequence. Statistical scores are computed to reduce false positive errors due to false alignments and sequence homology artifacts. This is followed by variant annotation-based frequency, mutation type, and other functional criteria. The combination filtering parameters along with inheritance modeling (if available) is then performed to narrow the number of causative mutations to a manageable number for further investigation. Knowledge databases (HGMD, OMIM) provide functional information that is helpful for interpretation. In clinical laboratories, potential causative variants are Sanger-confirmed and a report is generated after review

The third phase of analysis is the process of classifying the variants by utilizing NGS software and a number of knowledge databases (Fig. 8.1). Examples of biological, genomic, and mutation databases include OMIM (http://omim.org/) database, and locus-specific databases (LSDBs; http://www.hgvs.org/dblist/glsdb.html) and HGMD. For inheritance filtering, the method uses simple genotype comparison utilizing inheritance modeling between parents (plus other additional family members) and the proband. Multiple inheritance models, including autosomal-dominant, autosomal recessive, X-linked dominant, and X-linked recessive, are performed on the genotypes of the family members. For the autosomal recessive model, since there needs to be two affected alleles in the proband, variants that are homozygous or compound heterozygous (bi-allelic) in proband that are inherited from the parents are kept and move down the filtering pipeline. An advantage of having exome data for family members is that variants can be easily focused by this type of inheritance modeling filter. However, this requires data to be available for each family member adding to the cost and sometimes parental samples may not be readily available. Examples of commercially available software that performs inheritance modeling are NextGENe from SoftGenetics and SVS Suite from Golden Helix.

8.4.3.2   Inheritance Models for Autosomal Recessive Disorders: A Detailed Example

Autosomal recessive inheritance models can be directly applied to the family genotypes to filter out polymorphisms to obtain a smaller subset of potentially significant variants. It is possible that in the autosomal recessive model variants are homozygous (both inherited), compound heterozygous (both inherited), a combination of an inherited and a de novo variant, or two de novo variants. In the homozygous case, variants are heterozygous in parents and homozygous in the proband. To see if these variants fit this model, genotypes based on their genomic coordinates are compared to the parent in the NextGENe software. In the compound heterozygous model, the genotypes of parents can be easily sorted to further confirm the *trans* configuration of alleles. In the de novo and inherited model, the filtering of variants that are homozygous and compound heterozygous where one allele is inherited and the other de novo is performed. This type of comparison is different from the others in that genes found by de novo filtering must be compared to all the candidate variants. In the de novo case, parental genotypes are required to rule out transmission of variants. In this case, parents and unaffected siblings of the affected individual are negative for a specific genotype. Following variant annotation, candidate variants are further prioritized by functional filtering, namely, mutation types, presence of variants in mutation databases, frequency, predicted pathogenicity of variants, and case–control comparisons to remove background errors and match phenotypic description (Fig. 8.1).

8.4.4 Exome Sequencing Diagnostic Applications

The cost-effectiveness and usefulness of NGS-targeted panel designs for the diagnosis of genetic diseases, namely, hearing loss, muscular dystrophy, neuromuscular diseases, monogenic disease, cardiovascular diseases, retinitis pigmentosa, and mitochondrial disorders, have been shown numerous times and this diagnostic application of NGS is being extended to the analysis of exomes in clinical laboratories (Neveling et al. 2012; Vasli et al. 2012; Faita et al. 2012; Rehm 2013; Sivakumaran et al. 2013; Valencia et al. 2013; Wong 2013a; Treff et al. 2013). The genetic diagnosis of congenital chloride diarrhea in a patient was made through WES revealing a homozygous missense variant in *SLC26A3* (Choi et al. 2009). However, other studies have adopted whole genome sequencing (WGS) as a diagnostic application. For example, it was applied to an 11-month-old patient with severe hypercholesterolemia who was found to have mutations in *ABCG5* (Rios et al. 2010). Although WGS has been utilized for diagnostic applications, WES would have been sufficient to identify the causal variants and genes for severe hypercholesterolemia and the cost of a diagnostic test is an important consideration. WES is increasingly being utilized in molecular diagnosis (Bonnefond et al. 2010; Worthey et al. 2011).

8.4.5 Tiered Clinical Exome Analysis

In addition to performing primary, secondary, and tertiary analyses (Sect. 8.4.3.1) similar to research exomes, clinical exome analysis is a tiered approach to facilitate clinical interpretation of variants. The first step is to focus on genes (~5,000) with known disease associations and reported mutations. Genes found in the databases OMIM and HGMD are prioritized. Then, variants in genes (~15,000) with unknown phenotype or disease associations are screened as a second step. Unfortunately, this comprises a larger fraction of the exome. In some instances, the mode of inheritance may not be clear and all possible inheritance models must be processed. This increases the complexity of the test and may affect the turnaround time.

8.4.6 Clinical Exome Analysis Guided by Clinical Features

While there are over 20,000 known genes which are targeted by various capture kits, only about 5,000 genes have been associated with disease (OMIM and HGMD). Since functional interpretation of genes with unknown disease association is challenging, the clinical features of a case can be used to focus the search of causative variant(s) to genes with previously described associations. Various databases, such as the OMIM, provide gene lists and corresponding clinical features and disease associations. This focused approach may be another filter that can be used in

the analysis to narrow down the variants and increase the chance of finding causative variants. In addition, any potential causative variant has to be Sanger
sequencing-confirmed, the gold standard in clinical laboratories.

8.4.7   Clinical Laboratories Offering Exome Sequencing

The major genetic centers in the United States offering WES as a diagnostic test are
Cincinnati Children's Medical Center's Molecular Genetics Laboratory, Emory
Genetics Laboratory, Baylor College of Medicine, GeneDx, and Ambry Genetics.
Generally, the turnaround time of the exome test is between 10 and 16 weeks.
Pricing varies from $5,000 to $15,000 depending on the level of analysis and
whether only the proband or a trio is analyzed. For trio analysis, all laboratories
provide a report only for the proband. To aid in interpretation, a pedigree, patient
history, medical records, and clinical form are typically requested and some laboratories require this information before the test can be started. An extensive consent
form needs to be filled out prior to test commencement. To ensure the advantages
and limitations of the test are fully understood by the family members involved,
pre- and post-counseling is recommended. Generally, the Illumina HiSeq 2000/2500
sequencer and the NimbleGen capture are the platforms of choice for performing
this test in clinical laboratories.

8.4.8   Clinical Exome Data and Interpretation Challenges

There are various challenges that should be noted when performing exome assays
for a diagnostic purpose. The assay only covers between 90 and 97 % of the targeted
regions at a coverage level of 10X. This coverage depends on the type of capture
technology that is used with the key players in the field being NimbleGen, Illumina,
and Agilent Technologies (Su et al. 2011). In addition, many regions of the exome
remain unexplored and novel genes found in these locations have not yet been associated with disease. However, these gene regions cannot be ruled out in the analysis
and may require reanalysis of the data a year from the initial analysis to see if other
new disease associations are obtained (Klee et al. 2011). Another challenge of
exome analysis is that regions that play a role in regulating gene expression will not
be captured; expanded strategies such as genome will play a role in complementing
WES in this area. Alternatively, other exome capture products that include 5′ and 3′
UTR regions are starting to make their way into the marketplace. Due to the limited
size of the sequence reads of 100 bp, short sequence deletion and insertions (indels)
detection will be limited to about 1/3 of the read length. Larger indels will not be
detected for comprehensive mutation inclusion. This will improve by complementing assembly-like methods before alignment in a stepwise manner (Wong 2013b).
Furthermore, there are a high number of false positive findings for various reasons.

One source of errors can be attributed to the ambiguousness of the underlying sequence such as regions with high degree of similarity. Another reason for error calling is the incompleteness of the human reference sequence and the uncertainty degree of novel sequences. The ambiguity of the human reference sequence poses challenges for variant interpretations. A proper interpretation of sequence changes should be complemented by matched case–control testing. Novel associations require specialized knowledge of the disease mechanism and understanding of the proteins involved in the pathway. A heuristic approach to interpreting changes provides the means for personalized accurate interpretation.

8.5   Summary

Clinical WES has been shown to improve molecular diagnoses and alter patient management, as well as, provide identification of genes related to specific phenotypes to enhance functional research efforts (Yu et al. 2012; Coonrod et al. 2013). With the advent of enrichment methods and parallelized sequencing the cost of WES has recently decreased. More importantly, data management and interpretation tools have become more efficient in handling large amounts of data. Clinical WES also can improve diagnosis by determination of genetic causality and health care delivery for patients/families. We foresee the diagnostic use of WES to increase overtime and such information will enrich the SNP and mutation databases, thus, providing a step forward towards an improved description of the exome. The paradigm is shifting from single gene to WES in pediatrics, and medicine in general, and is the central theme of genomic medicine.

References

Abecasis GR, Altshuler D, Auton A et al (2010) A map of human genome variation from population-scale sequencing. Nature 467:1061–1073. doi:10.1038/nature09534

Birney E, Stamatoyannopoulos JA, Dutta A et al (2007) Identification and analysis of functional elements in 1% of the human genome by the ENCODE pilot project. Nature 447:799–816. doi:10.1038/nature05874

Bolze A, Byun M, McDonald D et al (2010) Whole-exome-sequencing-based discovery of human FADD deficiency. Am J Hum Genet. The American Society of Human Genetics. Elsevier, New York, pp 873–81

Bonnefond A, Durand E, Sand O et al (2010) Molecular diagnosis of neonatal diabetes mellitus using next-generation sequencing of the whole exome. PLoS One 5:e13630. doi:10.1371/journal.pone.0013630

Botstein D, Risch N (2003) Discovering genotypes underlying human phenotypes: past successes for mendelian disease, future approaches for complex disease. Nat Genet 33(Suppl):228–237. doi:10.1038/ng1090

Choi M, Scholl UI, Ji W et al (2009) Genetic diagnosis by whole exome capture and massively parallel DNA sequencing. Proc Natl Acad Sci U S A 106:19096–19101. doi:10.1073/pnas.0910672106

Coelho D, Kim JC, Miousse IR et al (2012) Mutations in ABCD4 cause a new inborn error of vitamin B12 metabolism. Nat Genet 44:1152–1155. doi:10.1038/ng.2386

Collin RWJ, Safieh C, Littink KW et al (2010) Mutations in C2ORF71 cause autosomal-recessive retinitis pigmentosa. Am J Hum Genet 86:783–788. doi:10.1016/j.ajhg.2010.03.016

Coonrod EM, Durtschi JD, Margraf RL, Voelkerding KV (2013) Developing genome and exome sequencing for candidate gene identification in inherited disorders: an integrated technical and bioinformatics approach. Arch Pathol Lab Med 137:415–433. doi:10.5858/arpa.2012-0107-RA

Dibbens LM, de Vries B, Donatello S et al (2013) Mutations in DEPDC5 cause familial focal epilepsy with variable foci. Nat Genet 45:546–551. doi:10.1038/ng.2599

Faita F, Vecoli C, Foffa I, Andreassi MG (2012) Next-generation sequencing in cardiovascular diseases. World J Cardiol 4:288–295. doi:10.4330/wjc.v4.i10.288

Gilissen C, Arts HH, Hoischen A et al (2010) Exome sequencing identifies WDR35 variants involved in Sensenbrenner syndrome. Am J Hum Genet 87:418–423. doi:10.1016/j.ajhg.2010.08.004

Harville HM, Held S, Diaz-Font A et al (2010) Identification of 11 novel mutations in eight BBS genes by high-resolution homozygosity mapping. J Med Genet 47:262–267. doi:10.1136/jmg.2009.071365

Hoischen A, van Bon BWM, Gilissen C et al (2010) De novo mutations of SETBP1 cause Schinzel-Giedion syndrome. Nat Genet 42:483–485. doi:10.1038/ng.581

Iseri SU, Wyatt AW, Nürnberg G et al (2010) Use of genome-wide SNP homozygosity mapping in small pedigrees to identify new mutations in VSX2 causing recessive microphthalmia and a semidominant inner retinal dystrophy. Hum Genet 128:51–60. doi:10.1007/s00439-010-0823-6

Johnson JO, Gibbs JR, Van Maldergem L et al (2010a) Exome sequencing in Brown-Vialetto-van Laere syndrome. Am J Hum Genet 87:567–569; author reply 569–570. doi:10.1016/j.ajhg.2010.05.021

Johnson JO, Mandrioli J, Benatar M et al (2010b) Exome sequencing reveals VCP mutations as a cause of familial ALS. Neuron 68:857–864. doi:10.1016/j.neuron.2010.11.036

Klee EW, Hoppman-Chaney NL, Ferber MJ (2011) Expanding DNA diagnostic panel testing: is more better? Expert Rev Mol Diagn 11:703–709. doi:10.1586/erm.11.58

Krawitz PM, Schweiger MR, Rödelsperger C et al (2010) Identity-by-descent filtering of exome sequence data identifies PIGV mutations in hyperphosphatasia mental retardation syndrome. Nat Genet 42:827–829. doi:10.1038/ng.653

Ku CS, Naidoo N, Pawitan Y (2011) Revisiting Mendelian disorders through exome sequencing. Hum Genet 129:351–370. doi:10.1007/s00439-011-0964-2

Lalonde E, Albrecht S, Ha KCH et al (2010) Unexpected allelic heterogeneity and spectrum of mutations in Fowler syndrome revealed by next-generation exome sequencing. Hum Mutat 31:918–923. doi:10.1002/humu.21293

Musunuru K, Pirruccello JP, Do R et al (2010) Exome sequencing, ANGPTL3 mutations, and familial combined hypolipidemia. N Engl J Med 363:2220–2227. doi:10.1056/NEJMoa1002926

Neveling K, Collin RW, Gilissen C et al (2012) Next-generation genetic testing for retinitis pigmentosa. Hum Mutat 33:963–972. doi:10.1002/humu.22045

Ng SB, Turner EH, Robertson PD et al (2009) Targeted capture and massively parallel sequencing of 12 human exomes. Nature 461:272–276. doi:10.1038/nature08250

Ng SB, Bigham AW, Buckingham KJ et al (2010a) Exome sequencing identifies MLL2 mutations as a cause of Kabuki syndrome. Nat Genet 42:790–793. doi:10.1038/ng.646

Ng SB, Buckingham KJ, Lee C et al (2010b) Exome sequencing identifies the cause of a mendelian disorder. Nat Genet 42:30–35. doi:10.1038/ng.499

Okou DT, Steinberg KM, Middle C et al (2007) Microarray-based genomic selection for high-throughput resequencing. Nat Methods 4:907–909. doi:10.1038/nmeth1109

Pang J, Zhang S, Yang P et al (2010) Loss-of-function mutations in HPSE2 cause the autosomal recessive urofacial syndrome. Am J Hum Genet 86:957–962

Pierce SB, Walsh T, Chisholm KM et al (2010) Mutations in the DBP-deficiency protein HSD17B4 cause ovarian dysgenesis, hearing loss, and ataxia of Perrault Syndrome. Am J Hum Genet 87:282–288. doi:10.1016/j.ajhg.2010.07.007

Rehm HL (2013) Disease-targeted sequencing: a cornerstone in the clinic. Nat Rev Genet 14: 295–300. doi:10.1038/nrg3463

Rios J, Stein E, Shendure J et al (2010) Identification by whole-genome resequencing of gene defect responsible for severe hypercholesterolemia. Hum Mol Genet 19:4313–4318. doi:10.1093/hmg/ddq352

Sivakumaran TA, Husami A, Kissell D et al (2013) Performance evaluation of the next-generation sequencing approach for molecular diagnosis of hereditary hearing loss. Otolaryngol–Head Neck Surg Off J Am Acad Otolaryngol-Head Neck Surg 148:1007–1016. doi: 10.1177/0194599813482294

Su Z, Ning B, Fang H et al (2011) Next-generation sequencing and its applications in molecular diagnostics. Expert Rev Mol Diagn 11:333–343. doi:10.1586/erm.11.3

Sulonen AM, Ellonen P, Almusa H et al (2011) Comparison of solution-based exome capture methods for next-generation sequencing. Genome Biol 12(9):R94

Tennessen JA, Bigham AW, O'Connor TD et al (2012) Evolution and functional impact of rare coding variation from deep sequencing of human exomes. Science 337:64–69. doi:10.1126/science.1219240

Treff NR, Fedick A, Tao X et al (2013) Evaluation of targeted next-generation sequencing-based preimplantation genetic diagnosis of monogenic disease. Fertil Steril 99:1377–1384.e6. doi:10.1016/j.fertnstert.2012.12.018

Valencia CA, Ankala A, Rhodenizer D et al (2013) Comprehensive mutation analysis for congenital muscular dystrophy: a clinical PCR-based enrichment and next-generation sequencing panel. PLoS One 8(1):e53083

Vasli N, Böhm J, Le Gras S et al (2012) Next-generation sequencing for molecular diagnosis of neuromuscular diseases. Acta Neuropathol (Berl) 124:273–283. doi:10.1007/s00401-012-0982-8

Walsh T, Shahin H, Elkan-Miller T et al (2010) Whole exome sequencing and homozygosity mapping identify mutation in the cell polarity protein GPSM2 as the cause of nonsyndromic hearing loss DFNB82. Am J Hum Genet 87:90–94. doi:10.1016/j.ajhg.2010.05.010

Wang JL, Yang X, Xia K et al (2010a) TGM6 identified as a novel causative gene of spinocerebellar ataxias using exome sequencing. Brain J Neurol 133:3510–3518. doi:10.1093/brain/awq323

Wang K, Li M, Hakonarson H (2010b) ANNOVAR: functional annotation of genetic variants from high-throughput sequencing data. Nucleic Acids Res 38(16):e164. doi:10.1093/nar/gkq603

Wheeler DL, Barrett T, Benson DA et al (2007) Database resources of the National Center for Biotechnology Information. Nucleic Acids Res 38:D5–16. doi:10.1093/nar/gkp967

Wong LJ (2013a) Next generation molecular diagnosis of mitochondrial disorders. Mitochondrion. doi:10.1016/j.mito.2013.02.001

Wong L-JC (2013b) Next generation molecular diagnosis of mitochondrial disorders. Mitochondrion 13:379–387. doi:10.1016/j.mito.2013.02.001

Worthey EA, Mayer AN, Syverson GD et al (2011) Making a definitive diagnosis: successful clinical application of whole exome sequencing in a child with intractable inflammatory bowel disease. Genet Med 13:255–262. doi:10.1097/GIM.0b013e3182088158

Yu Y, Wu BL, Wu J, Shen Y (2012) Exome and whole-genome sequencing as clinical tests: a transformative practice in molecular diagnostics. Clin Chem 58(11):1507–1509

Yu L, Wynn J, Cheung YH et al (2013) Variants in GATA4 are a rare cause of familial and sporadic congenital diaphragmatic hernia. Hum Genet 132:285–292. doi:10.1007/s00439-012-1249-0

Chapter 9
Challenges of Next-Generation–Sequencing-Based Molecular Diagnostics

9.1 Introduction

Although targeted sequencing by next-generation–sequencing (NGS) technology has gained much attention in the field of molecular diagnostics, several limitations have delayed its application to medical genetics. It is difficult to standardize the procedures because of the use of various sequencing platforms and target enrichment methods, which are updated rapidly. The cutoff thresholds for accurate variant identification, including the minimum read depth, range of variant percentage compared with the wild type, and quality score, have not been fully defined. Variable coverage depth across target regions and misalignment between homologous sequences or pseudogenes may also affect the accuracy of sequencing data. The fast falling sequencing cost and rapid development of NGS analyzing bioinformatics pipeline make it possible to use gene panels, whole exome sequencing (WES), and whole genome sequencing (WGS) for clinical diagnoses. However, there are many challenges in developing and implementing NGS technology for clinical use. Understanding these challenges can help molecular diagnostic professionals and ordering health professionals better gauge the utility of NGS clinical tests and the interpretation of the NGS results. NGS is a complex sequencing technology and many challenging steps need to be carried out to complete the test to generate clinically useful interpretations.

In this chapter, we will address the challenges of NGS technologies at various steps of the process including sample processing, data analyses, testing validation and revalidation, quality management of NGS testing, reporting and interpretation, informed consent and genetic counseling, training and education, and cost and reimbursement.

C.A. Valencia et al., *Next Generation Sequencing Technologies in Medical Genetics*,
SpringerBriefs in Genetics, DOI 10.1007/978-1-4614-9032-6_9,
© C. Alexander Valencia 2013

9.2   Sample Processing and Standardization of Capture and Sequencing Platforms

Sample processing for NGS is a much more complex process compared to Sanger sequencing. It typically includes DNA isolation, library generation, target enrichment, barcoding, and massive parallel sequencing (Mamanova et al. 2010). In addition, there are many new NGS platforms and chemistries that are being invented and introduced by different companies. Each capture and sequencing platform has its advantages and disadvantages. Unfortunately, clinical laboratories have not reached an agreement as to which technology is best for clinical testing, in part, because the technologies are new and keep rapidly improving. For example, the major suppliers for pre-sequencing library generation and target enrichment include SeqCap EZ Library series from NimbleGen-Roche, Nextera Rapid Capture Exome, TruSight Portfolio from Illumina, and SequalPrep and SOLiD Fragment Library Construction from Life Technologies.

Rapid adoption of the NGS technologies by clinical laboratories is often challenging because of the cost, validation time, specialized staff training, and lack of a sequencing instrument standard. Different types of sequencing chemistries are commercially available which include sequencing by synthesis, sequencing by ligation with reversible terminators, capture hybridization, and ion sensing (Glenn 2011). However, there is a lack of NGS instrument standard in clinical laboratories. Adopting such NGS technologies in clinical laboratories takes time because each sequencing chemistry requires its own instrument and the related purchasing cost, needs its own standard operation protocols (SOPs), generates its unique format of sequencing output, and the sequencing performance parameters must be established by extensive validation studies. Even the most seasoned medical technologists often have no NGS testing experience and it is the clinical laboratory's responsibility to provide costly and time-consuming training opportunities to be competent in handling patient samples for NGS clinical tests.

9.3   Data Analysis

Given the large amount of sequence data produced by NGS platforms, it is critical to have an efficient, reliable, and fast data handling and processing pipeline. When the sequencing is complete, sequence reads are aligned and analyzed against the consensus sequences and existing public databases (dbSNP and HGMD) to detect sequence variants. This requires extensive bioinformatics support and hardware infrastructure. In addition, the clinical laboratory must have its SOP to guarantee that the analytical pipeline can accurately track sample identity, particularly if barcoding is used. There are many challenges to assure the accuracy and reproducibility in data analyses. NGS data analysis can be divided into four basic steps: base calling, read alignment, variant calling, and variant annotation and filtering.

9.3.1   Base Calling

Each NGS platform has its own specific sequencing biases which could affect the types and rates of errors made during the data generation. These can include signal intensity decay over the read and erroneous insertions and deletions in homopolymeric stretches (Ledergerber and Dessimoz 2011). It is critical to utilize a base-calling package that is designed to reduce specific platform-related errors. Phred-like score associated with each base call (or other quality metric and measurement scores) is a useful measurement for the quality of platform-specific base calling.

9.3.2   Reads Alignment

Several commercially available or open-source tools (GATK and NextGENe) for read alignment are available which utilize a variety of alignment algorithms and may be more efficient for certain types of data than for others (Li and Homer 2010). They differ in accuracy and processing speed. Depending upon the types of variations expected, it is critical to choose one or more read alignment tools to be applied to the data. In addition, proper alignment can be challenging in the region with high homologous sequences, but it can be improved by longer or paired-end reads.

9.3.3   Variant Calling

The accuracy of variant calling depends on the depth of sequence coverage and the bi-direction reads of the sequences. Most variant calling algorithms are capable of detecting single or multiple base variations, while different algorithms may have more or less sensitivity to detect insertions and deletions (indels), large copy number variants (CNVs), and structural chromosomal rearrangements (translocations and inversions). Large deletions and duplications can be detected either by comparing actual read depth of a region to the expected read depth or through paired-end read mapping. Paired-end and mate-pair mapping can also be used to identify translocations and other structural rearrangements. However, it is recommended to confirm these results with microarray comparative genomic hybridization (aCGH), microarray CNVs, and other testing.

9.3.4   Variant Annotation and Filtering

Given the massive coverage of WES and WGS, WES identifies tens of thousands of variants while WGS identifies several millions. It is impossible to manually assess all variants in each patient. An automatic filtering approach must be applied for WES/WGS studies which may even need to be considered for large disease-targeted panels. Therefore, it is important to understand the variant filtering strategy to understand the sensitivity and limitations of test results. In addition, it is well-known that many databases contain misclassified variants, particularly benign variation misclassified as disease-causing (Bell et al. 2011). As a result, there are very few variant databases which are professionally curated to a clinical grade with evidence-based assessment of clinical and function data. In addition, most Mendelian diseases have a large percentage of variants that are private (unique to families) requiring a robust process for assessing novel variation and clinical laboratories that identified these mutations may not release the information via publications in a timely manner.

In the analysis of WES/WGS, common assumptions have to be made to set the algorithm for variant filtering, which include (1) causative mutations for Mendelian disorders are rare, (2) disease is highly penetrant, (3) mode of disease inheritance, and (4) phenotype-based filtering (Majewski et al. 2011). Successfully identifying the molecular basis for a rare disorder may depend on the strategy employed, such as availability of appropriate family members for comparison, given a suspected mode of inheritance. Regardless of the approach employed, it is recommended that referring physicians provide detailed phenotypic information to assist the clinical laboratory in analyzing and interpreting the results of testing. This step is a necessity for WES/WGS to enable appropriate filtering strategies to be employed. It is also highly recommended for large disease panel testing, given the diversity of genes and sub-phenotypes that may be included in a test panel. The ability for clinical laboratories to prioritize variants for further consideration or likely relevance may be dependent on the constellation of symptoms and findings in the patient (phenotype filter). However, physicians typically have very busy schedules and the complete clinical information may not be communicated at the time of requesting the test. A good practice is to follow up with the physician to complete the clinical inquiries prior to the data analyses. Clinical laboratories must set thresholds to balance over-filtering that could inadvertently exclude causative variants with under-filtering that presents too many variants for farther analyses. Clinical laboratories should provide a summary of the variant filtering strategy to assist ordering healthcare professionals to understand the sensitivity and specificity of the test results.

9.4   Testing Validation and Revalidation

Various combinations of instruments, reagents, and analytical pipelines may be used in tests involving NGS. The entire test should be validated using allowed sample types before clinical laboratory implementation. Assay performance characteristics including analytical sensitivity and specificity as well as the assay's repeatability and reproducibility need to be established (Mattocks et al. 2010). For a clinical laboratory, the initial setup for an NGS test could be very burdensome; however, it is necessary to go through this process to understand the benefit and limitation of NGS tests to provide clinical interpretations with confidence. For WES/WGS, the focus of validation is shifted more towards developing metrics that define a high quality exome/genome such as the average coverage across the exome/genome and the percentage of bases that meet a set minimum coverage threshold. An evaluation of the concordance of SNPs identified compared to the reference should be made for WES. In practice, this may entail sequencing a larger number of samples to cover sufficient numbers of variants. Several clinical laboratories have used 95–98 % concordance as the minimum acceptable level. In addition, homologous sequences such as pseudogenes pose a challenge for all short read sequencing approaches. The limited length of NGS sequence reads can lead to false positive variant calls when reads are incorrectly aligned to a homologous region, but also to false negative results when variant-containing reads align to homologous loci. Therefore, the clinical laboratory must develop a strategy for detecting disease-causing variants within regions with known homology in its validation protocol. Rescue or conformational testing may be warranted based on the indication and the specificity of the test defined by the laboratory. Test development costs, analytical sensitivity and specificity, and analysis complexity are important factors that must be evaluated when considering development of NGS services. An ongoing QC monitoring of NGS testing is also critical given the fast development of the testing and analyzing strategies to ensure quality results. Any major change of testing protocol should be thoughtfully revalidated before implementing it for clinical service. The clinical laboratory should inform ordering health providers with these changes on a timely manner.

9.5   Quality Management of Next-Generation–Sequencing Testing

Multiple commercial NGS platforms have been developed, all of which have the capacity to sequence millions of DNA fragments in parallel. Differences in the sequencing chemistry of each platform result in differences in total sequence capacity, sequence read length, sequence run time, and final quality and accuracy of the data. These characteristics may influence the choice of platform to be used for a specific clinical application. The clinical laboratory must develop quality control (Q/C) measures and apply these to every run. These can vary depending on the chosen methods and sequencing instrument but typically include measures to identify sample preparation failures as well as measures to identify failed sequencing runs. The clinical laboratory must also track sample identity throughout the testing process, which is especially important given that NGS testing commonly entails pooling of barcoded samples. Proficiency testing protocols must also be established and executed periodically according to CLIA and CAP regulations.

9.6   Reporting and Interpretation

Disease-related gene panel testing is relatively straightforward in terms of reporting and interpretation. Sanger confirmation is used as complementary testing to "rescue" missing data from bases or regions that are not supported by a sufficient number of reads to confidently call variants. For disease-specific targeted panels, the clinical laboratory should establish the estimated clinical sensitivity of the test based upon a combination of analytical performance parameters and the known contribution of the targeted set of genes and types of variants detectable for that disease. In contrast, reporting for WES is very challenging. Currently, the best NGS tests can only cover 90–95 % of the targeted exome (Cirulli et al. 2010). WGS covers both coding and noncoding regions. Due to limitations in the interpretation of noncoding variants, coding regions are often analyzed first. For WES/WGS and certain large gene panels, it is acceptable to report results without complete coverage at a predefined minimum. The clinical laboratory director typically uses his/her discretion to judge the need for Sanger sequencing to fill-in missing areas of a test. Therefore, additional metrics that may be helpful for determining data quality include the percentage of reads aligned to the human genome, the percentage of bases corresponding to targeted sequences, and the percentage of targeted bases with no coverage. For WES/WGS of patients with undiagnosed disorders, it is typically not feasible to calculate a theoretical clinical sensitivity for the test given its dependency on the applications and indications for testing. However, empirical data from one recent study suggests that these tests have a clinical sensitivity of approximately 24 % (Gahl et al. 2012). Long term, each clinical laboratory should track and share success rates across different disease areas to aid in setting realistic expectations for the likelihood of an etiology being detected for certain types of indications.

One strategy some clinical laboratories are adopting is to perform WES, but proceed with the interpretation of only genes already known to be disease-associated. This will post great challenge to estimate the sensitivity and specificity of these "panel" tests. It is the responsibility of the clinical laboratory to clarify the test methodology in the report for this type of testing, which is critical information to understand a "no mutation found" case and proceed to genetic counseling.

9.7   Informed Consent and Genetic Counseling

Pre- and posttest genetic counseling are essential steps for patients and their families to understand the implication with NGS-based testing. Unlike other genetic tests, NGS-based testing is more complex and the implications of the test results may not be as straightforward. Findings generated from these tests from different clinical laboratories using different technologies may have different implications for the patients and their family. For example, test results may reveal nonpaternity and other secondary findings that may change the clinical care for the patient and other family members. In this way, the ordering provider will be aware of the potential scope of incidental findings before ordering WES/WGS testing and can ensure that informed consent and shared decision-making with the patient includes a discussion of how incidental findings will be handled. Any return of incidental findings should be done in collaboration with the ordering provider to ensure those results are interpreted in the context of the patient's medical and family history and personal desires for receiving incidental results. Genetic counseling should be offered to these patients prior and after the NGS tests.

Gene discovery has historically been limited to research laboratories. This is now changing with the ability to perform WES/WGS to identify novel disease gene candidates in the clinical laboratory. Therefore, it is critical for a clinical laboratory to have an informed consent in place to offer further studies, often in collaboration with research laboratories, to prove the disease association. In addition, if no mutation that can explain the patient's symptoms is identified, the data can be reanalyzed for the remaining WES/WGS potential to identify new disease gene associations which would be beyond the capacity of a clinical test.

9.8   Training and Education

Given the technical and interpretive complexity of NGS, it is recommended by ACMG that the reporting and oversight of clinical NGS-based testing be performed by individuals with appropriate professional training and certification (American Board of Medical Genetics-certified medical/laboratory geneticists or American Board of Pathology-certified molecular genetic pathologists) and with extensive experience in the evaluation of sequence variation and evidence for disease causation as well as technical expertise in sequencing technologies. For clinical laboratories offering WES services, they should have access to broad clinical genetics expertise for evaluating the relationships between genes, variation, and disease phenotypes. Finding people with the correct education and certification to perform the WES/WGS testing is another challenge that many clinical laboratories have to face. Ongoing training is necessary to keep up with this fast developing field.

9.9   Cost and Reimbursement

NGS provides a massive information output at a relatively low cost; however, it is still cost-prohibitive to many families if such test is not covered by their health insurance or government program (e.g., Medicare/Medicaid). Depending on the scale of the testing, the price for NGS ranges from several thousands to tens of thousands of dollars. The American economy is still in the face of recovering from the recent recession. The record high of national debt will affect the government funding for healthcare and healthcare research for many years to come. In addition, currently (March 2013) there is no specific CPT code, generated by the American

Medical Association, for NGS tests. Therefore, it is valuable to have a pre-certification process in place to work with physician on this issue and to engage the private payer and government agencies to understand the NGS role in improving patient care.

9.10   Summary

NGS makes it possible to identify disease etiologies for genetic conditions with substantial genetic heterogeneity and to identify novel disease-causing mutations and novel disease associate genes. However, clinical laboratories need to overcome many technical, economical, and ethical obstacles to make it a viable tool for clinical diagnosis.

References

Bell CJ, Dinwiddie DL, Miller NA et al (2011) Carrier testing for severe childhood recessive diseases by next-generation sequencing. Sci Transl Med 3:65ra4. doi:10.1126/scitranslmed.3001756

Cirulli ET, Singh A, Shianna KV et al (2010) Screening the human exome: a comparison of whole genome and whole transcriptome sequencing. Genome Biol 11:R57. doi:10.1186/gb-2010-11-5-r57

Gahl WA, Markello TC, Toro C et al (2012) The National Institutes of Health Undiagnosed Diseases Program: insights into rare diseases. Genet Med 14:51–59. doi:10.1038/gim.0b013e318232a005

Glenn TC (2011) Field guide to next-generation DNA sequencers. Mol Ecol Resour 11:759–769. doi:10.1111/j.1755-0998.2011.03024.x

Ledergerber C, Dessimoz C (2011) Base-calling for next-generation sequencing platforms. Brief Bioinform 12:489–497. doi:10.1093/bib/bbq077

Li H, Homer N (2010) A survey of sequence alignment algorithms for next-generation sequencing. Brief Bioinform 11:473–483. doi:10.1093/bib/bbq015

Majewski J, Schwartzentruber J, Lalonde E et al (2011) What can exome sequencing do for you? J Med Genet 48:580–589. doi:10.1136/jmedgenet-2011-100223

Mamanova L, Coffey AJ, Scott CE et al (2010) Target-enrichment strategies for next-generation sequencing. Nat Methods 7:111–118. doi:10.1038/nmeth.1419

Mattocks CJ, Morris MA, Matthijs G et al (2010) A standardized framework for the validation and verification of clinical molecular genetic tests. Eur J Hum Genet 18:1276–1288. doi:10.1038/ejhg.2010.101